The Breathwork Path

Techniques for Mind and Body Harmony

www.xspurts.com

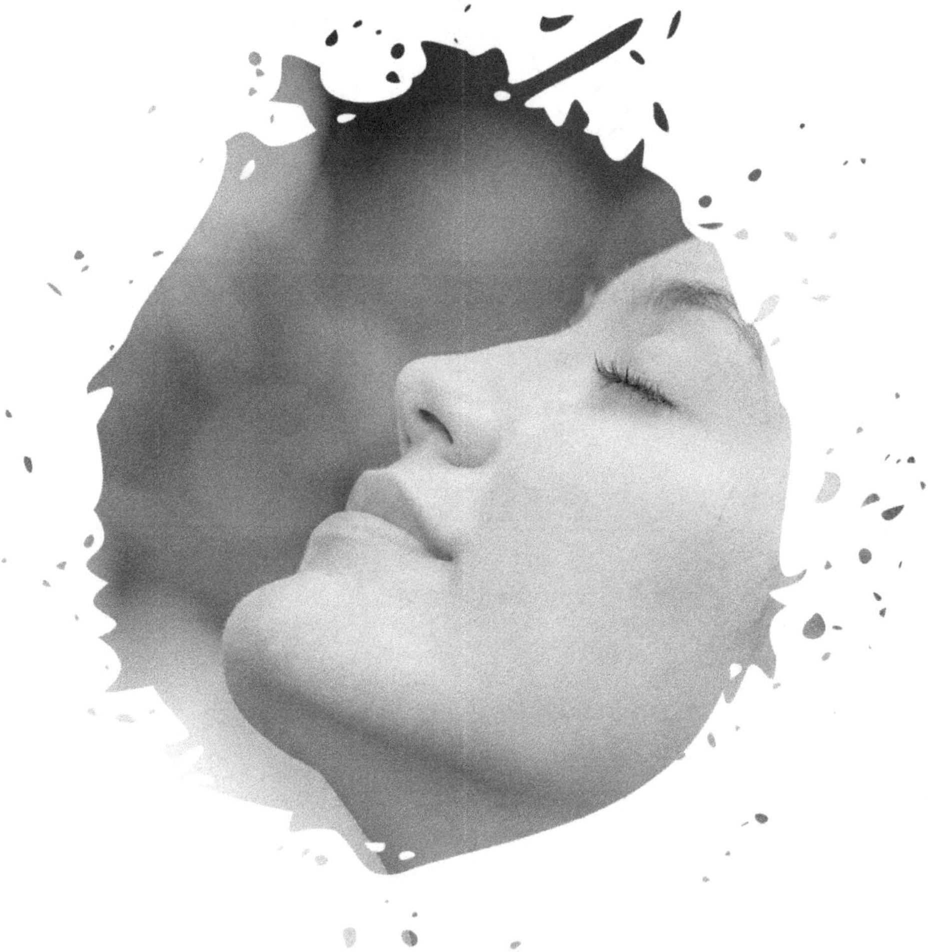

Get A Free Book At: xspurts.com/posts/free-book-offer

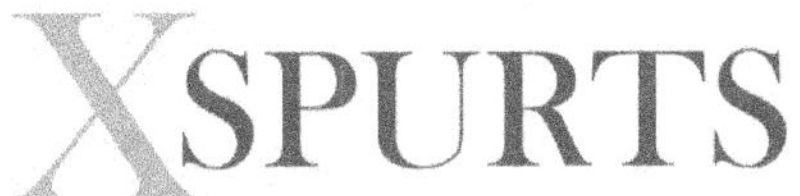

Table of Contents

The Essence of Breathwork

The Essence of Breathwork

Breathwork is a practice that has been gaining popularity in recent years for its profound effects on physical, mental, and emotional well-being. It is a therapeutic technique that involves conscious control and manipulation of the breath to promote relaxation, reduce stress, and enhance overall health. In this essay, we will delve into the essence of breathwork, exploring its history, techniques, and the numerous benefits it offers.

Historical Roots:

Breathwork is not a new concept; it has ancient roots in various cultures and traditions around the world. Practices like Pranayama in yoga, Qigong in Chinese medicine, and Tummo in Tibetan Buddhism all involve intentional breath control for healing and spiritual purposes. These practices have been passed down through generations, emphasizing the importance of the breath in achieving balance and vitality.

Techniques and Approaches:

There are several breathwork techniques and approaches, each with its unique focus and benefits. Some of the most common include:

Diaphragmatic Breathing: This technique emphasizes deep breathing, engaging the diaphragm to maximize oxygen intake and release toxins. It is a fundamental practice that forms the basis of many other breathwork techniques.

Box Breathing: Box breathing, also known as square breathing, involves inhaling, holding, exhaling, and holding the breath in equal counts. It helps calm the nervous system, reduce anxiety, and improve focus.

Holotropic Breathwork: Developed by Dr. Stanislav Grof, holotropic breathwork is a powerful method for accessing altered states of consciousness. It involves rapid and deep breathing to release emotional and psychological blockages.

Wim Hof Method: Created by "The Iceman" Wim Hof, this method combines specific breathing techniques with cold exposure and meditation to enhance physical and mental performance, boost the immune system, and reduce stress.

Pranayama: Pranayama is a collection of breathing exercises in yoga that can range from calming and grounding to energizing and purifying. It is a fundamental aspect of yoga practice, helping to balance the body and mind.

Benefits of Breathwork:

Breathwork offers a wide range of benefits for individuals seeking improved well-being. Some of the key advantages include:

Stress Reduction: One of the most immediate and noticeable benefits of breathwork is stress reduction. Deep, controlled breathing activates the body's relaxation response, reducing cortisol levels and promoting a sense of calm.

Improved Mental Clarity: Breathwork enhances mental clarity and focus by increasing oxygen flow to the brain. This can help individuals think more clearly, make better decisions, and boost productivity.

Emotional Release: Breathwork can release pent-up emotions and traumas stored in the body. It provides a safe space for individuals to process and heal emotional wounds.

Enhanced Physical Health: Practicing breathwork regularly can improve lung capacity, increase energy levels, and support overall physical health. It also aids in detoxification by expelling waste and toxins from the body.

Better Sleep: Breathwork can improve sleep quality by calming the mind and reducing nighttime anxiety. Many people find that incorporating breathwork into their bedtime routine leads to more restful sleep.

Spiritual Growth: For some, breathwork serves as a spiritual practice, providing a pathway to heightened states of consciousness and self-discovery. It can lead to a deeper connection with oneself and the universe.

Accessibility and Inclusivity:

One of the remarkable aspects of breathwork is its accessibility and inclusivity. Unlike some wellness practices that require specific equipment or environments, breathwork can be done anywhere and by anyone. It is a practice that transcends age, gender, and physical abilities, making it a valuable tool for improving the well-being of a wide range of individuals.

In conclusion, the essence of breathwork lies in its ability to harness the power of the breath to improve physical, mental, and emotional health. With a rich history rooted in ancient traditions and a diverse array of techniques, breathwork offers a holistic approach to well-being that is accessible to all. Whether used as a tool for stress reduction, mental clarity, emotional release, or spiritual growth, breathwork has the potential to transform lives and foster a deeper connection to oneself and the world around us.

Understanding Breathwork

Understanding Breathwork

Breathwork, often referred to as a powerful tool for self-improvement and well-being, has gained significant recognition in recent years. This practice, rooted in ancient traditions and adapted for modern lifestyles, involves conscious control and manipulation of the breath to achieve various physical, mental, and emotional benefits. In this essay, we will delve into the fascinating world of breathwork, exploring its origins, techniques, and the profound impact it can have on one's life.

Historical Roots:

Breathwork is not a new concept but has been practiced in various forms for centuries across different cultures and traditions. Its origins can be traced back to ancient practices such as Pranayama in yoga, Qigong in Chinese medicine, and Tummo in Tibetan Buddhism. These practices recognized the vital role of breath in achieving balance, vitality, and spiritual growth. Over time, these ancient techniques have evolved and adapted to contemporary needs.

Techniques and Approaches:

Breathwork encompasses a wide range of techniques and approaches, each with its unique focus and intended benefits. Some of the most prevalent techniques include:

Diaphragmatic Breathing: This fundamental technique emphasizes deep, slow breaths that engage the diaphragm. It is often the starting point for those new to breathwork, helping individuals become more aware of their breath and its impact on their state of being.

Box Breathing: Box breathing, also known as square breathing, involves inhaling, holding, exhaling, and holding the breath for equal counts. This practice helps regulate the autonomic nervous system, promoting relaxation and reducing stress.

Holotropic Breathwork: Developed by Dr. Stanislav Grof, holotropic breathwork is a technique designed to access altered states of consciousness. Participants engage in rapid and deep breathing to release emotional and psychological blockages, often leading to profound insights and healing.

Wim Hof Method: Created by Wim Hof, also known as "The Iceman," this method combines specific breathing techniques, cold exposure, and meditation. It aims to boost physical and mental performance, enhance the immune system, and reduce stress.

Pranayama: In yoga, Pranayama encompasses a variety of breathing exercises that range from calming and grounding to energizing and purifying. These practices are integral to the yoga tradition, promoting balance and overall well-being.

Benefits of Breathwork:

Breathwork offers a multitude of benefits that can positively impact one's physical, mental, and emotional health. Some of the key advantages include:

Stress Reduction: One of the most immediate and noticeable benefits of breathwork is its ability to reduce stress. Conscious breathing activates the body's relaxation response, lowering cortisol levels and promoting a sense of calm.

Enhanced Mental Clarity: Breathwork increases oxygen flow to the brain, improving mental clarity and focus. This can aid individuals in making better decisions and increasing productivity.

Emotional Release: Breathwork can serve as a powerful tool for emotional release. By consciously engaging with the breath, individuals can access and process deep-seated emotions and traumas, leading to healing and inner peace.

Improved Physical Health: Regular breathwork practices can enhance lung capacity, increase energy levels, and support overall physical health. It also aids in detoxification by facilitating the removal of waste and toxins from the body.

Better Sleep: Breathwork can improve sleep quality by calming the mind and reducing nighttime anxiety. Many individuals find that incorporating breathwork into their bedtime routine leads to more restful sleep.

Spiritual Growth: For some, breathwork is a gateway to spiritual exploration and personal growth. It can facilitate a deeper connection with one's inner self and the universe, fostering a sense of interconnectedness.

Accessibility and Inclusivity:

One of the remarkable aspects of breathwork is its accessibility and inclusivity. Unlike some wellness practices that require specific equipment or environments, breathwork can be practiced anywhere and by anyone. It transcends age, gender, and physical abilities, making it a valuable tool for improving the well-being of a diverse range of individuals.

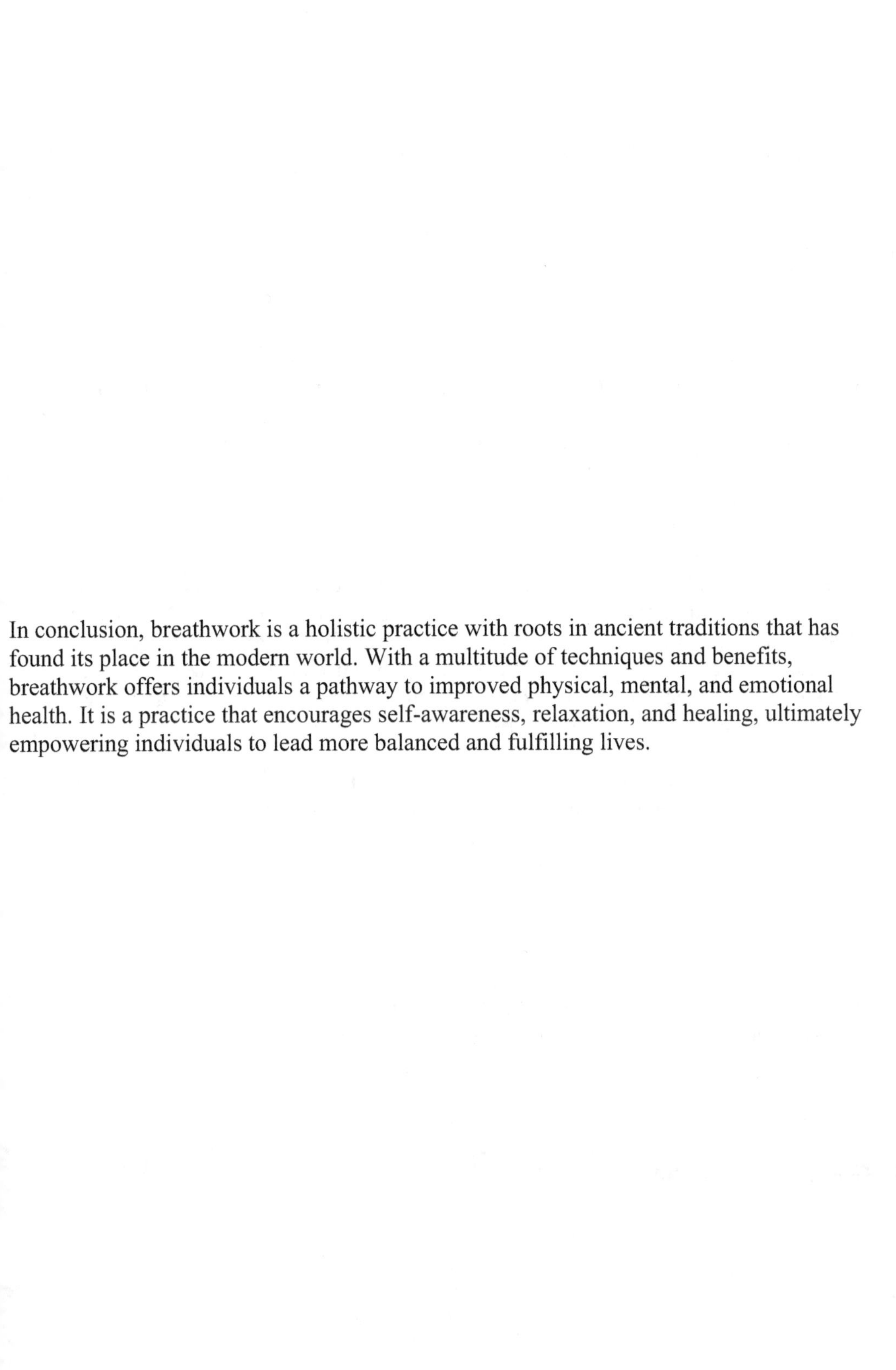

In conclusion, breathwork is a holistic practice with roots in ancient traditions that has found its place in the modern world. With a multitude of techniques and benefits, breathwork offers individuals a pathway to improved physical, mental, and emotional health. It is a practice that encourages self-awareness, relaxation, and healing, ultimately empowering individuals to lead more balanced and fulfilling lives.

Historical Perspectives on Breathing Practices

Historical Perspectives on Breathing Practices

Breathing is a fundamental and involuntary act that sustains life. Throughout history, various cultures and civilizations have recognized the significance of breath and developed practices to harness its power for physical, mental, and spiritual well-being. These historical perspectives on breathing practices provide valuable insights into the origins and evolution of breathwork.

Ancient Civilizations:

The roots of breathwork can be traced back to ancient civilizations that understood the profound connection between breath and life force. In ancient India, the practice of Pranayama was developed as an integral component of yoga. Pranayama involves the conscious control and regulation of the breath to enhance physical vitality and spiritual growth. It is documented in ancient texts like the Upanishads and the Yoga Sutras of Patanjali, dating back over 2,000 years.

In China, the philosophy of Qi (or Chi) emphasized the flow of vital energy through the body. Qigong, a practice that combines breath control, meditation, and movement, aimed to balance and harmonize this energy. Qigong's origins can be traced back over 4,000 years to the ancient Chinese dynasties.

Ancient Greece:

Ancient Greek philosophers also recognized the significance of breath. The term "pneuma" was used to describe the vital breath or life force. Philosophers like Aristotle and Diogenes emphasized the connection between breath and the mind, believing that the quality of one's breath influenced one's thoughts and emotions.

Hippocrates, often regarded as the father of modern medicine, recognized the importance of balanced breathing for health. He advocated for deep and rhythmic breathing to maintain physical and mental well-being.

Medieval and Renaissance Europe:

During the Middle Ages, breathing practices were incorporated into various religious and mystical traditions. Christian mystics engaged in contemplative practices that involved controlled breathing to deepen their connection with the divine. The Desert Fathers, a group of early Christian hermits, practiced controlled breathing as a means of spiritual purification.

In the Renaissance period, the concept of "spiritus" (Latin for breath) gained prominence. It was believed that the breath carried the essence of life and vitality. This era saw the revival of interest in ancient Greek and Roman philosophies, which included a renewed focus on the relationship between breath, mind, and body.

Modern Developments:

As the scientific understanding of human physiology advanced, so did the exploration of breathing practices. In the early 20th century, Russian scientist Konstantin Buteyko developed the Buteyko Method, which aimed to treat various respiratory conditions through breathing exercises. His work laid the foundation for contemporary breathwork practices.

In the 20th and 21st centuries, influential figures like Dr. Herbert Benson introduced the "Relaxation Response," highlighting the physiological benefits of deep and rhythmic breathing in reducing stress. Moreover, pioneers like Dr. Stanislav Grof developed holotropic breathwork as a means of accessing altered states of consciousness and facilitating psychological healing.

Conclusion:

Historical perspectives on breathing practices reveal a rich tapestry of cultural and philosophical beliefs surrounding the significance of breath. These practices have evolved over millennia, from ancient India and China to Greece and beyond, reflecting the enduring human fascination with the breath's potential to enhance physical, mental, and spiritual well-being.

Today, breathwork continues to evolve, with diverse techniques and approaches that cater to the needs and interests of individuals worldwide. The historical wisdom and insights into the power of breath serve as a foundation for the contemporary practice of breathwork, offering a holistic approach to health and inner transformation.

Fundamentals of Breathing

Fundamentals of Breathing

Breathing is an essential and automatic bodily function that provides oxygen to our cells and removes carbon dioxide, allowing us to survive. However, beyond its life-sustaining role, breathing has a profound impact on our physical and mental well-being. Understanding the fundamentals of breathing is crucial, particularly in the context of breathwork, a practice that harnesses the power of breath to enhance health and inner harmony.

Mechanics of Breathing:

Breathing is a complex process involving the coordination of multiple muscles and the expansion and contraction of the lungs. The primary muscles responsible for breathing are the diaphragm, intercostal muscles, and various accessory muscles.

- Diaphragm: The diaphragm is a dome-shaped muscle that separates the chest cavity from the abdominal cavity. When it contracts, it flattens and moves downward, creating a vacuum in the chest, which draws air into the lungs. This is known as inhalation.

- Intercostal Muscles: These muscles, located between the ribs, assist in expanding the chest cavity during inhalation and contracting during exhalation.

- Accessory Muscles: These muscles, including those in the neck and shoulders, come into play during deep or rapid breathing, such as during physical exertion.

Breathing Patterns:

Normal breathing typically involves a rhythmic pattern known as "respiratory sinus arrhythmia," characterized by a slight increase in heart rate during inhalation and a decrease during exhalation. This pattern is associated with relaxation and emotional regulation.

However, various factors, such as stress, anxiety, or physical exertion, can disrupt this pattern, leading to shallow, rapid breathing. In contrast, deep and diaphragmatic breathing, also known as "belly breathing," involves slower, more deliberate breaths that engage the diaphragm. This type of breathing is associated with relaxation and reduced stress.

The Role of Carbon Dioxide:

One crucial aspect of breathing is the balance of oxygen and carbon dioxide in the blood. While oxygen is essential for cellular function, carbon dioxide plays a vital role in regulating pH levels in the blood. When we inhale oxygen, it is transported to our cells, where it participates in energy production. In return, our cells produce carbon dioxide as a metabolic waste product.

The body carefully maintains a balance between oxygen and carbon dioxide levels. If we overbreathe, as in cases of rapid or shallow breathing, we expel too much carbon dioxide, which can lead to symptoms like dizziness, tingling sensations, and even panic. Breathwork practices often focus on restoring this balance by emphasizing slower, deeper breaths that allow for optimal oxygenation while retaining an appropriate level of carbon dioxide.

Breathing and the Autonomic Nervous System:

Breathing is intimately connected to the autonomic nervous system (ANS), which regulates involuntary bodily functions, including heart rate, digestion, and respiratory rate. The ANS has two branches: the sympathetic nervous system (SNS), responsible for the "fight or flight" response, and the parasympathetic nervous system (PNS), associated with the "rest and digest" state.

Slow, deep breathing, such as the kind practiced in breathwork, stimulates the PNS, promoting relaxation, reducing stress, and lowering heart rate. Conversely, shallow, rapid breathing activates the SNS, leading to heightened alertness and increased heart rate.

Conclusion:

The fundamentals of breathing go beyond mere oxygen exchange; they influence our physiological and psychological states. Breathwork, as a practice, leverages these fundamentals to enhance well-being, reduce stress, and promote emotional and physical balance. By understanding the mechanics of breathing, the role of carbon dioxide, and its connection to the autonomic nervous system, individuals can harness the power of their breath to cultivate a deeper sense of inner calm and vitality.

Anatomy of Breathing

Anatomy of Breathing

Breathing is a fundamental and often overlooked aspect of our daily lives, but its anatomy is both intricate and essential. Understanding the anatomy of breathing is crucial in the practice of breathwork, a holistic approach to health and well-being that leverages the power of breath to promote physical and mental harmony.

The Respiratory System:

At the core of breathing is the respiratory system, a complex network of organs and tissues responsible for the exchange of oxygen and carbon dioxide in the body. Key components of the respiratory system include:

Nose and Mouth: The process of breathing begins with the inhalation of air through the nose or mouth. These openings filter, humidify, and warm the incoming air, making it suitable for the respiratory passages.

Pharynx and Larynx: Air passes through the pharynx and larynx, where the vocal cords are located. The larynx also prevents food and drink from entering the airway during swallowing.

Trachea: The trachea, often referred to as the windpipe, is a tube that carries air from the larynx to the bronchi. It is reinforced with C-shaped cartilage rings to keep it open and prevent collapse.

Bronchi and Bronchioles: The trachea divides into two bronchi, which further branch into smaller bronchioles. These airways lead to the alveoli, where gas exchange occurs.

Alveoli: The alveoli are tiny, air-filled sacs at the end of bronchioles. They are surrounded by capillaries and serve as the site for the exchange of oxygen and carbon dioxide between the lungs and the bloodstream.

Lungs: The lungs are the primary organs of respiration. They consist of lobes (left lung has two, right lung has three) and are enclosed by the pleura, a double-layered membrane that helps protect and maintain lung function.

Diaphragm: The diaphragm is a thin, dome-shaped muscle that separates the chest cavity from the abdominal cavity. It plays a crucial role in the mechanics of breathing. When it contracts, it flattens and moves downward, increasing the volume of the chest cavity during inhalation.

The Mechanics of Breathing:

The act of breathing involves a complex interplay of muscles and changes in pressure within the chest cavity. There are two main phases of breathing:

Inhalation: During inhalation, the diaphragm contracts and moves downward, creating a vacuum in the chest cavity. This action causes the chest to expand, and the lungs fill with air as the air pressure inside the lungs becomes lower than the atmospheric pressure.

Exhalation: Exhalation is a passive process in which the diaphragm relaxes and moves upward. This reduces the volume of the chest cavity, increasing the air pressure in the lungs. As a result, air is expelled from the lungs.

The Role of Accessory Muscles:

While the diaphragm is the primary muscle involved in breathing, other muscles can come into play during deep or forceful breaths. Accessory muscles, including those in the neck and shoulders, assist in expanding the chest cavity further, enabling deeper breaths when needed, such as during physical exertion.

The Influence of Posture:

Posture also plays a significant role in the mechanics of breathing. An upright and balanced posture allows for optimal lung expansion and diaphragmatic function. Poor posture, on the other hand, can restrict the movement of the diaphragm and lead to shallow breathing.

Breathing and the Autonomic Nervous System:

The autonomic nervous system (ANS) regulates involuntary bodily functions, including breathing. The ANS comprises two branches: the sympathetic nervous system (SNS) and the parasympathetic nervous system (PNS).

- SNS: The SNS is responsible for the "fight or flight" response and can increase the rate and depth of breathing to prepare the body for action.

- PNS: The PNS, on the other hand, is associated with the "rest and digest" state and promotes slower, deeper breathing, which is calming and helps reduce stress.

Understanding the anatomy of breathing is essential for individuals looking to explore breathwork and its potential benefits. Breathwork practices often focus on optimizing the mechanics of breathing to promote relaxation, reduce stress, and enhance overall well-being. By gaining insight into how the respiratory system works, individuals can make conscious efforts to harness the power of their breath and achieve a deeper sense of physical and mental harmony.

The Breath-Mind Connection

The Breath-Mind Connection

Breathing is a fundamental physiological function, but its significance extends far beyond mere survival. The way we breathe has a profound impact on our mental and emotional states, and this connection between breath and mind lies at the heart of breathwork, a holistic approach to well-being. In this essay, we'll explore the intricate relationship between breath and the mind, shedding light on how conscious breathing techniques can positively influence our mental and emotional health.

The Mind-Body Nexus:

To understand the breath-mind connection, it's essential to recognize the intimate link between the mind and the body. Our mental and emotional states can have a direct impact on our breathing patterns, and conversely, our breath can influence our mental and emotional well-being.

Stress and Shallow Breathing:

One of the most common manifestations of this connection is observed during times of stress and anxiety. When we experience stress, our body's fight-or-flight response is triggered, leading to rapid, shallow breathing. This type of breathing restricts the flow of oxygen to the brain, which can exacerbate feelings of anxiety and panic. It becomes a vicious cycle—stress influences breathing, and shallow breathing intensifies stress.

Breath as a Tool for Stress Reduction:

Conversely, we can use our breath as a powerful tool to mitigate stress and anxiety. By practicing conscious, deep breathing techniques, we can activate the body's relaxation response through the parasympathetic nervous system. This promotes a sense of calm and can help alleviate stress and anxiety symptoms.

Mindful Breathing:

One of the foundational principles of breathwork is mindfulness, which involves paying deliberate attention to each breath as it enters and leaves the body. Mindful breathing allows us to anchor our awareness to the present moment, reducing rumination on past or future events that often lead to stress and anxiety.

Breath Retention and Mental Clarity:

Certain breathwork practices incorporate breath retention techniques, where the breath is held for a specific duration. These practices are believed to enhance mental clarity, focus, and concentration. They stimulate the brain and increase oxygen levels, creating an alert and clear mental state.

Emotional Release:

Breathwork can also serve as a vehicle for emotional release. Many individuals carry unresolved emotions within them, which can manifest as physical tension or mental distress. Breathwork practices often involve deep, rhythmic breathing that can help release stored emotions, providing a sense of relief and catharsis.

Regulating Emotions:

Incorporating conscious breathing into daily life can assist in emotional regulation. By taking slow, deep breaths when faced with challenging emotions, individuals can create a space for reflection and response rather than reacting impulsively. This emotional regulation can lead to more balanced and harmonious relationships with oneself and others.

Enhancing Mind-Body Coordination:

Breathwork practices that synchronize breath with movement, such as yoga and tai chi, promote enhanced mind-body coordination. These practices require focused attention on breath patterns while moving through postures or sequences, fostering a deeper connection between physical and mental awareness.

The Power of Intention:

Intention is a vital aspect of breathwork. By setting specific intentions for a breathwork session, individuals can harness the breath to achieve their desired mental and emotional states. Whether it's cultivating gratitude, finding inner peace, or reducing stress, the breath becomes a tool for manifesting intentions.

In conclusion, the breath-mind connection is a profound and intricate relationship that underscores the principles of breathwork. Through conscious breathing techniques, individuals can harness the power of the breath to positively influence their mental and emotional well-being. By cultivating mindfulness, regulating emotions, and setting intentions, breathwork offers a holistic approach to achieving a state of balance and harmony between the mind and body. Ultimately, it reminds us that the breath is not just

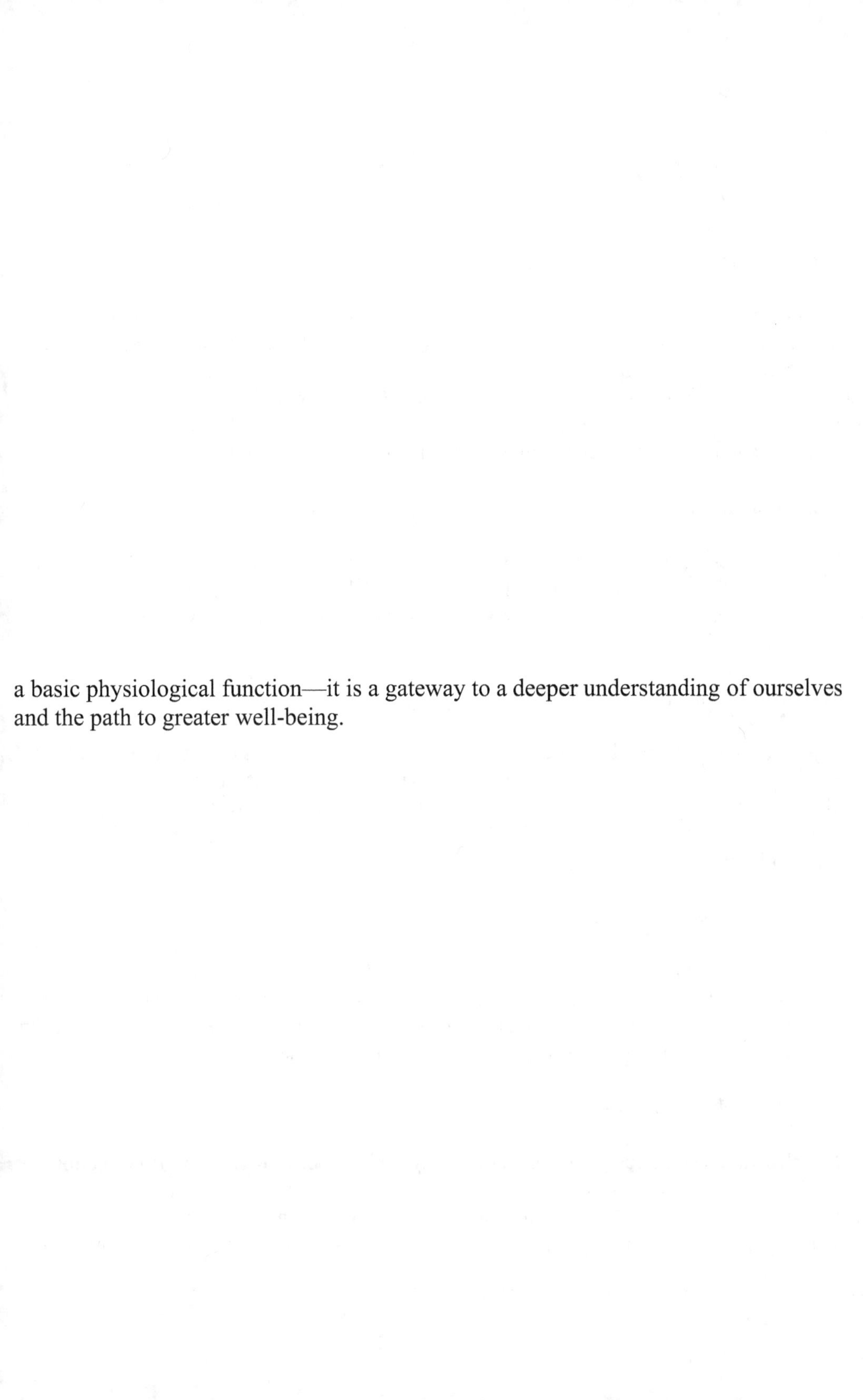

a basic physiological function—it is a gateway to a deeper understanding of ourselves and the path to greater well-being.

Breath Awareness Exercises

Breath Awareness Exercises

Breathwork is a holistic practice that involves conscious control and awareness of one's breath to promote physical, mental, and emotional well-being. Within the realm of breathwork, breath awareness exercises hold a special place. These exercises focus on observing and understanding one's breath without necessarily altering it. In this essay, we'll delve into the significance of breath awareness exercises and explore how they contribute to a greater understanding of the breath-mind connection.

Observing the Natural Breath:

Breath awareness exercises begin with a simple premise: observing the natural breath as it flows in and out without attempting to change it. This practice encourages individuals to become keen observers of their breath patterns and the sensations associated with breathing.

Present-Moment Awareness:

One of the fundamental benefits of breath awareness exercises is their ability to cultivate present-moment awareness. In a world filled with distractions and constant mental chatter, these exercises anchor individuals to the here and now. By focusing on the breath, individuals can develop mindfulness, which is the practice of being fully present without judgment.

Reducing Stress and Anxiety:

Stress and anxiety often manifest in erratic and shallow breathing patterns. By engaging in breath awareness exercises, individuals can become aware of these patterns and work towards restoring natural, deep breaths. This shift from shallow to deep breathing triggers the body's relaxation response, reducing stress and anxiety levels.

Enhancing Mind-Body Connection:

Breath awareness exercises also foster a stronger mind-body connection. By directing attention to the breath, individuals can perceive how their mental and emotional states impact their breathing patterns. For example, moments of tension or anxiety may lead to shallow breathing, while feelings of relaxation may result in deeper, slower breaths. This heightened awareness promotes self-reflection and the ability to consciously influence one's state of being.

Recognizing Breath Holding:

Many individuals unknowingly hold their breath during stressful or challenging situations. Breath awareness exercises shed light on this tendency, helping individuals recognize when they are holding their breath and why. This awareness can serve as a valuable tool for breaking the habit of breath-holding and encouraging continuous, rhythmic breathing.

Balancing the Autonomic Nervous System:

The autonomic nervous system regulates involuntary bodily functions, including breathing. Breath awareness exercises can contribute to the balance of this system by promoting coherence between the sympathetic (fight-or-flight) and parasympathetic (rest-and-digest) branches. This balance is essential for overall well-being.

Enhancing Concentration and Focus:

Focused attention on the breath is a central element of breath awareness exercises. This sustained concentration can spill over into other areas of life, enhancing an individual's ability to concentrate and maintain focus, whether at work, in sports, or during daily activities.

Self-Regulation:

Breath awareness exercises empower individuals to self-regulate their emotional and mental states. By recognizing how different emotions influence their breath, individuals can take proactive steps to regulate these emotions. For instance, they can consciously slow their breathing when faced with anger or anxiety, leading to a calmer state of mind.

Complementary to Other Breathwork Practices:

Breath awareness exercises complement other breathwork practices, such as deep breathing techniques, breath retention, or guided visualizations. They serve as a foundational practice that deepens an individual's understanding of their breath and enhances their ability to engage in more advanced breathwork.

In conclusion, breath awareness exercises play a crucial role in breathwork and holistic well-being. By simply observing the natural breath without trying to change it, individuals can cultivate mindfulness, reduce stress, enhance mind-body connection, and develop self-regulation skills. These exercises are accessible to anyone and can be incorporated into daily life to promote a greater understanding of the breath-mind connection. Ultimately, breath awareness exercises empower individuals to harness the transformative power of their breath for improved physical, mental, and emotional health.

Techniques of Breathwork

Techniques of Breathwork

Breathwork encompasses a diverse array of techniques and practices aimed at harnessing the power of breath to enhance physical, mental, and emotional well-being. From ancient yogic traditions to contemporary therapeutic modalities, breathwork techniques have evolved and adapted over time. In this essay, we will explore some of the most prominent and effective techniques of breathwork.

Diaphragmatic Breathing (Abdominal Breathing): Diaphragmatic breathing is a foundational breathwork technique that emphasizes deep, rhythmic breathing by engaging the diaphragm. This technique involves expanding the abdomen during inhalation and allowing it to contract during exhalation. Diaphragmatic breathing encourages the full utilization of lung capacity and is known for its calming effect on the nervous system.

Box Breathing (Square Breathing): Box breathing is a structured breathwork technique that involves equalizing the duration of inhalation, breath retention, exhalation, and another breath retention, typically in a 4-4-4-4 pattern. This technique can promote relaxation, reduce stress, and enhance focus and concentration.

Pranayama: Pranayama is a vast category of breathwork techniques originating from the ancient practice of yoga. These techniques involve specific breath patterns, such as Ujjayi (victorious) breath, Kapalabhati (skull-shining) breath, and Nadi Shodhana (alternate nostril) breath. Pranayama aims to balance the body's energy, enhance vitality, and promote mental clarity.

Holotropic Breathwork: Developed by Dr. Stanislav Grof, holotropic breathwork is a transformative technique that combines rapid, deep breathing with evocative music and bodywork. This technique is used for self-exploration, emotional healing, and accessing altered states of consciousness. It is often practiced in a group setting under the guidance of a trained facilitator.

Buteyko Breathing Method: The Buteyko method is a breathwork technique designed to correct chronic hyperventilation, which is believed to contribute to various health issues. Practitioners of this method learn to reduce the volume of their breath and increase carbon dioxide levels in the body, which can have a calming and stabilizing effect.

Transformational Breath: Transformational Breath is a contemporary breathwork modality that combines conscious connected breathing with body mapping and sound therapy. It aims to release physical and emotional tension, facilitate personal growth, and improve overall well-being. Practitioners often experience a sense of expanded awareness and emotional release.

Wim Hof Method: Developed by "The Iceman" Wim Hof, this technique combines specific breathing exercises with cold exposure and meditation. The method is known for its potential to increase energy, boost the immune system, and improve mental focus. It has gained popularity for its adaptogenic effects on the body.

4-7-8 Breathing: This breathwork technique involves inhaling for a count of 4, holding the breath for a count of 7, and exhaling for a count of It is often used as a relaxation exercise and can help individuals fall asleep more easily by calming the nervous system.

Circular Breathing: Circular breathing is a technique used by musicians, particularly wind instrument players, to maintain a continuous stream of air while playing. It involves inhaling through the nose while simultaneously exhaling through the mouth, allowing for uninterrupted music production.

Breath Retention (Kumbhaka): Breath retention is a component of various breathwork practices, including pranayama and holotropic breathwork. It involves voluntarily holding the breath after inhalation or exhalation for varying durations. Breath retention can induce altered states of consciousness and promote self-discovery.

In conclusion, breathwork encompasses a rich tapestry of techniques that cater to diverse needs and objectives. From traditional practices like pranayama to modern approaches like the Wim Hof Method, breathwork offers a versatile toolkit for enhancing physical health, mental clarity, emotional balance, and spiritual growth. These techniques empower individuals to explore the transformative potential of their own breath, leading to profound insights and a deeper connection to their inner selves. Whether used for relaxation, healing, personal growth, or spiritual exploration, breathwork continues to be a valuable and accessible resource for holistic well-being.

Basic Breathwork Techniques

Basic Breathwork Techniques

Breathwork, an ancient practice with roots in various spiritual and healing traditions, has gained popularity in recent years for its potential to enhance physical, mental, and emotional well-being. While there are numerous advanced breathwork techniques, mastering the basics is essential for those new to the practice. In this essay, we will explore some fundamental breathwork techniques that anyone can use to experience immediate benefits.

Diaphragmatic Breathing (Abdominal Breathing): Diaphragmatic breathing is one of the simplest and most foundational breathwork techniques. It involves breathing deeply into the diaphragm, allowing the abdomen to expand on inhalation and contract on exhalation. To practice diaphragmatic breathing, sit or lie down in a comfortable position. Place one hand on your chest and the other on your abdomen. Inhale slowly through your nose, feeling your abdomen rise, and then exhale through your mouth, feeling it fall. Focus on making your abdominal breath slow, deep, and rhythmic. This technique helps reduce stress and promotes relaxation.

4-7-8 Breathing: The 4-7-8 breathing technique is a simple yet effective way to calm the nervous system and reduce anxiety. To practice, sit or lie down comfortably. Close your eyes and take a deep breath in through your nose for a count of 4 seconds. Hold your breath for a count of 7 seconds, and then exhale completely through your mouth for a count of 8 seconds. Repeat this cycle for a few minutes, gradually extending the duration if comfortable. This technique can be used before bedtime to aid in falling asleep or during moments of stress for quick relief.

Box Breathing (Square Breathing): Box breathing is a structured breathwork technique that helps improve focus, reduce anxiety, and increase mindfulness. It involves equalizing the duration of inhalation, breath retention, exhalation, and another breath retention, typically in a 4-4-4-4 pattern. To practice, sit in a relaxed position and close your eyes. Inhale through your nose for a count of 4, hold your breath for a count of 4, exhale through your mouth for a count of 4, and then hold your breath again for a count of Repeat this cycle several times. Box breathing can be a valuable tool for enhancing concentration and managing stress.

Counted Breaths: Counted breaths is a simple technique that fosters mindfulness and relaxation. Find a quiet place to sit or lie down. Close your eyes and take a few natural breaths to settle in. Begin counting each inhalation and exhalation, starting at 1 and going up to When you reach 10, start over. If your mind wanders or you lose count, simply return to 1 and continue. This technique helps anchor your attention to the present moment and can be practiced for as long as you like.

Nostril Breathing: Nostril breathing, or alternate nostril breathing, is a pranayama technique from yoga that balances the flow of energy in the body and calms the mind. Sit comfortably and close your eyes. Use your right thumb to close your right nostril and inhale deeply through your left nostril. Then, use your right ring finger to close your left nostril while releasing the right nostril, and exhale completely. Continue by inhaling through the right nostril, then closing the right nostril again and exhaling through the left. Repeat this cycle for several rounds. Nostril breathing is excellent for centering and balancing the mind.

In conclusion, mastering basic breathwork techniques is a valuable first step for those looking to explore the benefits of this ancient practice. Whether you're seeking stress relief, improved focus, better sleep, or enhanced mindfulness, these fundamental techniques provide a solid foundation. Over time, you can explore more advanced breathwork practices and incorporate them into your daily routine for continued growth and well-being. Breathwork offers a simple yet profound way to tap into the power of your breath and cultivate a deeper connection with your inner self.

Advanced Pranayama Practices

Advanced Pranayama Practices

Pranayama, the ancient yogic practice of breath control, goes beyond basic breathing exercises and delves into advanced techniques that offer profound physical, mental, and spiritual benefits. These practices have been developed and refined over centuries, and they require patience, dedication, and guidance. In this essay, we will explore some advanced pranayama practices that can elevate your breathwork journey.

Kapalabhati (Skull-Shining Breath): Kapalabhati is a dynamic and invigorating pranayama technique that cleanses the respiratory system, energizes the body, and focuses the mind. To practice, sit in a comfortable position with your spine straight. Take a deep inhalation and then forcefully exhale through your nostrils by contracting your abdominal muscles. The inhalation should be passive and natural. Start with a few rounds of 30 rapid exhalations, gradually increasing the count as you become more comfortable. Kapalabhati should be practiced on an empty stomach and can be a refreshing way to start the day.

Nadi Shodhana (Alternate Nostril Breathing): Nadi Shodhana is a pranayama practice that balances the flow of energy in the body and calms the nervous system. Sit comfortably with your spine straight and close your eyes. Using your right thumb and ring finger, alternate closing and opening your nostrils. Start by closing your right nostril with your thumb and inhaling deeply through the left nostril. Then, close the left nostril with your ring finger and exhale through the right nostril. Inhale through the right nostril, close it, and exhale through the left nostril. Continue this cycle for several minutes. Nadi Shodhana is renowned for its ability to bring clarity and reduce stress.

Bhastrika (Bellows Breath): Bhastrika is a forceful and energizing pranayama practice that increases vitality and heats the body. To practice, sit comfortably and close your eyes. Take a deep inhalation through your nostrils, then forcefully exhale by contracting your abdominal muscles. The inhalation should be passive and natural. Practice rapid, rhythmic breaths, inhaling and exhaling through your nostrils. Start with 30 seconds and gradually increase the duration as you become more adept. Bhastrika can be an effective way to warm up before yoga or other physical activities.

Ujjayi (Ocean Breath): Ujjayi pranayama involves creating a soft, ocean-like sound in the throat while breathing, and it is often used during yoga practice to cultivate focus and internal heat. Begin by sitting or lying down comfortably. Inhale deeply through your nostrils, and as you exhale, constrict the muscles at the back of your throat to create a gentle, audible "haaah" sound. This sound should be continuous and even on both inhalation and exhalation. Ujjayi breath helps synchronize movement and breath during yoga, promoting mindfulness and relaxation.

Surya Bhedana (Right Nostril Breathing): Surya Bhedana is a pranayama technique that is believed to increase the body's energy and warmth. Sit comfortably and close your eyes. Using your right thumb, close your left nostril, and inhale deeply through your right nostril. Then, close the right nostril with your ring finger, release the left nostril, and exhale through the left. This constitutes one round. Continue for several rounds, focusing on the heat generated within your body. Surya Bhedana is often practiced during colder seasons to boost internal warmth.

Chandra Bhedana (Left Nostril Breathing): Chandra Bhedana is the opposite of Surya Bhedana and is believed to have cooling and calming effects on the body and mind. Sit comfortably and close your eyes. Using your ring finger, close your left nostril, and inhale deeply through your right nostril. Then, close the right nostril with your thumb, release the left nostril, and exhale through the left. This completes one round. Continue for several rounds, experiencing the soothing qualities of Chandra Bhedana. It can be practiced to calm the mind before meditation or sleep.

In conclusion, advanced pranayama practices offer a deeper exploration of the profound benefits of breathwork. While these techniques can be immensely rewarding, it's essential to approach them with caution and seek guidance from an experienced teacher if you're new to advanced pranayama. Regular practice of these techniques can enhance physical vitality, mental clarity, and spiritual connection, contributing to a more balanced and harmonious life. The journey of pranayama is a voyage of self-discovery and inner transformation, guided by the wisdom of the breath.

Breathwork for Relaxation and Stress Relief

Breathwork for Relaxation and Stress Relief

In today's fast-paced world, where stress and anxiety often take center stage, the simple act of conscious breathing can be a powerful tool for relaxation and stress relief. This practice, known as breathwork, offers numerous benefits for both the mind and body. In this essay, we will explore how breathwork can help you find tranquility, reduce stress, and enhance your overall well-being.

Understanding Breathwork:

Breathwork is a holistic practice that focuses on intentional control of the breath to achieve specific physical, mental, and emotional outcomes. It encompasses various techniques, each with its unique purpose and approach. The common thread among these techniques is the emphasis on conscious, deliberate breathing.

Stress and the Breath:

Stress and anxiety often manifest as shallow, rapid breathing. When we encounter stressful situations, our sympathetic nervous system activates the "fight or flight" response, leading to increased heart rate and shallow breathing. This response is essential for survival in the face of immediate danger, but chronic stress can lead to ongoing physiological imbalances.

Breathwork for Stress Reduction:

Deep Diaphragmatic Breathing: One of the simplest and most effective breathwork techniques for stress reduction is deep diaphragmatic breathing. To practice, find a quiet space, sit or lie down comfortably, and place one hand on your chest and the other on your abdomen. Inhale deeply through your nose, allowing your abdomen to rise as your diaphragm contracts. Exhale slowly through your mouth, feeling your abdomen fall. Focus on making your exhalations longer than your inhalations. This practice activates the parasympathetic nervous system, promoting relaxation and reducing stress.

Box Breathing: Box breathing, also known as square breathing, is a technique that helps regulate the breath and calm the mind. Start by inhaling through your nose for a count of four seconds, then hold your breath for four seconds, exhale for four seconds, and hold your breath again for four seconds before beginning the cycle anew. This pattern creates a square, and repeating it for several minutes can reset your nervous system and alleviate stress.

Progressive Muscle Relaxation: This breathwork technique combines conscious breathing with muscle relaxation. Begin by sitting or lying down and taking a few deep breaths to center yourself. Then, focus your attention on different muscle groups, starting from your toes and working your way up to your head. As you inhale, tense each muscle group, and as you exhale, release the tension. This practice helps you become more aware of bodily sensations and can effectively reduce physical and mental tension.

Guided Breathwork and Meditation: Many meditation and breathwork apps and videos are available, offering guided sessions specifically designed for relaxation and stress relief. These resources can be valuable tools for those looking to incorporate breathwork into their daily routines.

The Science Behind It:

Breathwork's effectiveness in reducing stress and promoting relaxation is supported by scientific research. When practiced regularly, conscious breathing can lower cortisol levels, reduce blood pressure, improve heart rate variability, and enhance overall well-being. These physiological changes contribute to a calmer and more relaxed state of mind.

In Conclusion:

Breathwork is a valuable practice that offers an accessible and effective way to combat stress and anxiety. By incorporating simple breathwork techniques into your daily routine, you can tap into the power of your breath to find relaxation, reduce stress, and improve your overall quality of life. Whether you choose deep diaphragmatic breathing, box breathing, progressive muscle relaxation, or guided breathwork and meditation, the key is consistency. Regular practice of breathwork can help you build resilience against life's stressors and promote a greater sense of inner calm and balance. So take a deep breath, exhale, and start your journey toward relaxation and stress relief through the power of breathwork.

Breathwork for Health and Wellness

Breathwork for Health and Wellness

In recent years, breathwork has gained increasing recognition for its potential to promote health and wellness. This ancient practice, rooted in various traditions and cultures, focuses on conscious control of the breath to enhance physical, mental, and emotional well-being. From reducing stress to improving lung function, breathwork offers a myriad of benefits that can positively impact your overall health. In this essay, we will delve into the science and techniques behind breathwork and explore its potential to enhance your health and wellness.

The Science Behind Breathwork:

Understanding the science behind breathwork is essential to grasp how it contributes to health and wellness. When we consciously control our breath, we influence the autonomic nervous system, which regulates involuntary bodily functions. Breathwork techniques can stimulate the parasympathetic nervous system, responsible for the "rest and digest" response, promoting relaxation and reducing stress. On the other hand, it can also engage the sympathetic nervous system, responsible for the "fight or flight" response, which can boost alertness and energy levels.

Benefits of Breathwork for Health and Wellness:

Stress Reduction: Chronic stress can take a toll on both mental and physical health. Breathwork techniques, such as deep diaphragmatic breathing and box breathing, activate the relaxation response, leading to reduced cortisol levels and a greater sense of calm.

Improved Lung Function: Many breathwork practices focus on expanding lung capacity and optimizing breathing patterns. These exercises can enhance oxygen exchange in the body, potentially improving lung function and overall respiratory health.

Enhanced Mental Clarity: Conscious breathing can sharpen focus, increase mental clarity, and boost cognitive performance. This can be particularly beneficial for tasks that require sustained attention and concentration.

Emotional Regulation: Breathwork encourages awareness of emotions and sensations in the body. This heightened awareness can aid in emotional regulation, helping individuals manage difficult emotions and cultivate a more balanced emotional state.

Better Sleep: Practicing breathwork before bedtime can calm the mind and relax the body, potentially leading to improved sleep quality. By reducing stress and anxiety, breathwork can help alleviate insomnia and sleep disturbances.

Pain Management: Some breathwork techniques, such as the Lamaze method, have been utilized for pain management during childbirth. These practices can also be adapted to manage chronic pain conditions by increasing pain tolerance and reducing the perception of discomfort.

Breathwork Techniques for Health and Wellness:

Pranayama: Pranayama is a yogic breathwork practice that encompasses various techniques, including Ujjayi (victorious) breath, Kapalabhati (skull-shining) breath, and Nadi Shodhana (alternate nostril) breath. Each technique has specific benefits, from calming the mind to balancing energy.

Holotropic Breathwork: Developed by psychiatrist Stanislav Grof, Holotropic Breathwork involves deep, rapid breathing to induce altered states of consciousness. This practice is often used for personal growth and spiritual exploration.

Wim Hof Method: Named after the "Iceman" Wim Hof, this method combines specific breathing techniques with cold exposure and meditation. It is known for boosting the immune system, increasing energy, and reducing stress.

Buteyko Breathing: Developed by Russian physician Konstantin Buteyko, this technique focuses on reducing overbreathing and promoting nasal breathing. It is often used to address respiratory conditions such as asthma.

Incorporating Breathwork into Your Wellness Routine:

To harness the benefits of breathwork for health and wellness, consider integrating it into your daily routine. Start with simple practices like deep diaphragmatic breathing, and gradually explore more advanced techniques as you become more comfortable. Many apps and online resources offer guided breathwork sessions to assist you on your journey to better health and well-being.

In conclusion, breathwork is a versatile and accessible tool for enhancing health and wellness. By understanding the science behind breathwork and exploring various techniques, you can unlock its potential to reduce stress, improve lung function, enhance mental clarity, regulate emotions, and more. Whether you're seeking relaxation, better sleep, or improved overall health, breathwork can be a valuable addition to your wellness toolkit. So take a deep breath, exhale, and embark on a path to greater health and well-being through the power of conscious breathing.

Breathwork in Physical Health Management

Breathwork in Physical Health Management

Breathwork, a practice that involves conscious control of the breath, has gained recognition for its potential to improve physical health and well-being. While breathwork has deep roots in ancient traditions and cultures, its relevance in modern physical health management is becoming increasingly apparent. In this essay, we will explore the ways in which breathwork contributes to physical health, from enhancing lung function to aiding in pain management.

Optimizing Lung Function:

One of the fundamental aspects of breathwork is optimizing lung function. Many individuals have inefficient breathing patterns, often characterized by shallow chest breathing. Such patterns can limit the amount of oxygen that reaches the cells and tissues of the body. Breathwork techniques, such as diaphragmatic breathing, encourage deep and controlled breaths that engage the diaphragm muscle. This practice increases lung capacity and the exchange of oxygen and carbon dioxide, leading to improved respiratory health.

Aiding in Respiratory Conditions:

Breathwork can be particularly beneficial for individuals with respiratory conditions such as asthma and chronic obstructive pulmonary disease (COPD). Techniques like Buteyko breathing, which emphasizes nasal breathing and reducing overbreathing, can help manage the symptoms of these conditions. By controlling the breath, individuals with respiratory issues can reduce the frequency and severity of attacks and improve overall lung function.

Pain Management and Tension Release:

Breathwork is often used as a complementary approach to pain management. Techniques like the Lamaze method, commonly used during childbirth, involve rhythmic breathing to reduce the perception of pain. Similar practices can be adapted to manage chronic pain conditions, such as fibromyalgia or lower back pain. By increasing pain tolerance and promoting relaxation, breathwork can serve as a valuable tool in physical therapy and pain relief.

Enhancing Athletic Performance:

Athletes have long recognized the potential benefits of breathwork in optimizing performance. Controlled and focused breathing can enhance endurance, improve oxygen utilization, and reduce the build-up of lactic acid in muscles. Techniques like the Wim Hof Method, which combines specific breathing practices with cold exposure, have gained popularity among athletes for their potential to boost energy levels and improve recovery.

Stress Reduction and Immune System Support:

Chronic stress can have a detrimental impact on physical health, weakening the immune system and contributing to various health problems. Breathwork techniques, especially those that activate the relaxation response, help reduce stress levels. This, in turn, supports immune system function and overall well-being. Practices like the Wim Hof Method have been associated with increased resistance to illnesses and improved immune response.

Blood Pressure Regulation:

High blood pressure, or hypertension, is a common health concern that can lead to serious cardiovascular problems. Breathwork, particularly practices involving slow, deep breaths, can help regulate blood pressure. When performed regularly, these techniques can contribute to maintaining healthy blood pressure levels and reducing the risk of heart-related issues.

Improved Digestion:

Breathwork can also play a role in digestive health. Deep, diaphragmatic breathing promotes relaxation and activates the parasympathetic nervous system, which is responsible for the "rest and digest" response. By reducing stress and tension, breathwork can aid in digestion and alleviate symptoms of gastrointestinal discomfort.

Incorporating breathwork into your physical health management routine can be a valuable step toward overall well-being. Whether you are seeking to optimize lung function, manage respiratory conditions, alleviate pain, enhance athletic performance, or reduce stress, breathwork offers a versatile and accessible tool. With various techniques available and resources such as guided sessions and mobile apps, integrating breathwork into your daily life has never been easier.

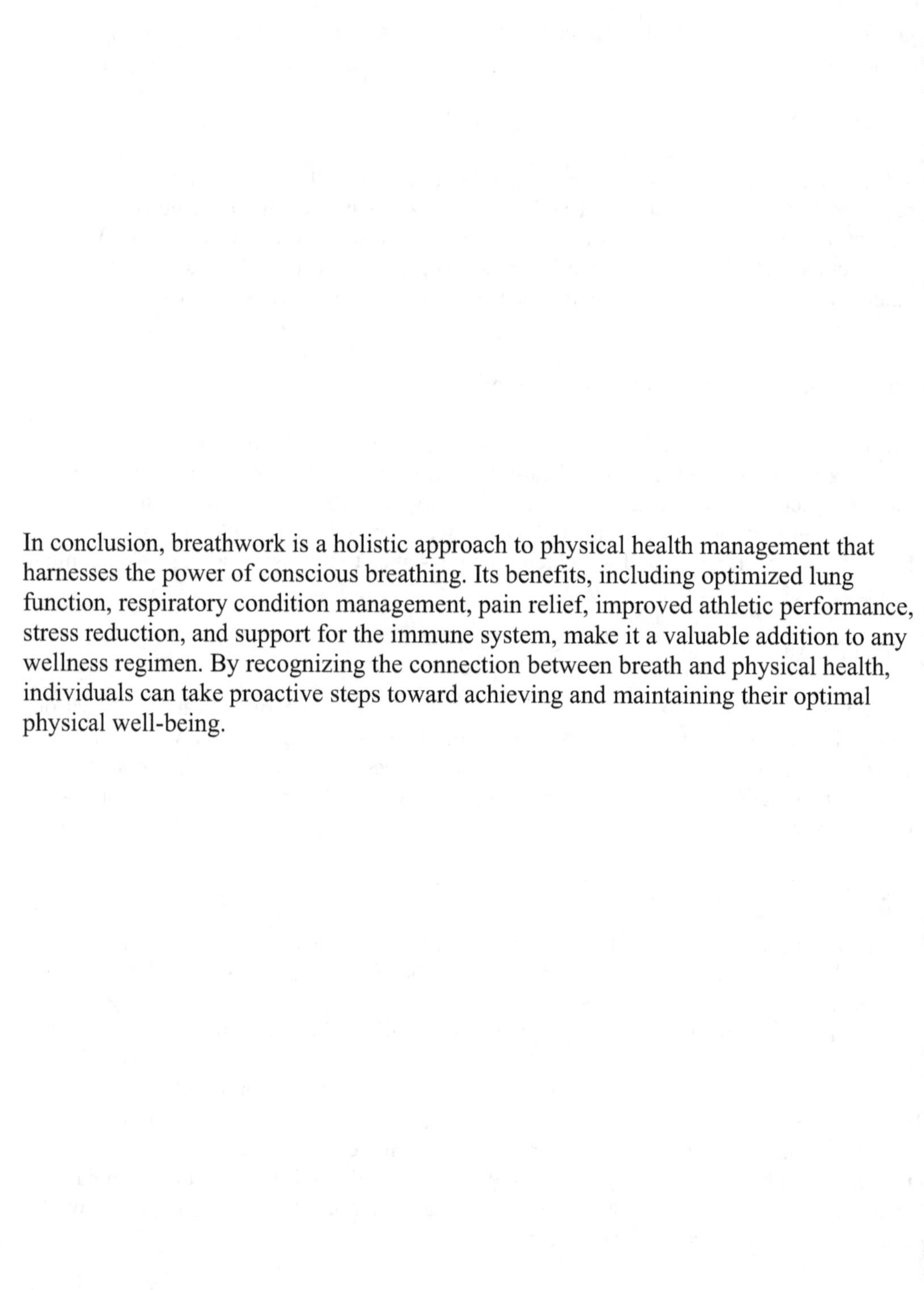

In conclusion, breathwork is a holistic approach to physical health management that harnesses the power of conscious breathing. Its benefits, including optimized lung function, respiratory condition management, pain relief, improved athletic performance, stress reduction, and support for the immune system, make it a valuable addition to any wellness regimen. By recognizing the connection between breath and physical health, individuals can take proactive steps toward achieving and maintaining their optimal physical well-being.

Breathwork for Mental and Emotional Well-being

Breathwork for Mental and Emotional Well-being

In the pursuit of mental and emotional well-being, individuals often explore a variety of practices and techniques. One such practice that has gained significant recognition in recent years is breathwork. Breathwork involves conscious control and manipulation of the breath to achieve various mental and emotional benefits. In this essay, we will delve into the ways in which breathwork can contribute to enhancing mental and emotional well-being.

Stress Reduction and Relaxation:

One of the most prominent benefits of breathwork for mental and emotional well-being is its ability to reduce stress and induce relaxation. Deep, intentional breathing activates the body's parasympathetic nervous system, responsible for the "rest and digest" response. This counteracts the effects of the sympathetic nervous system, which triggers the body's stress response. As a result, individuals who practice breathwork regularly experience reduced stress levels, leading to a greater sense of calm and relaxation.

Anxiety Management:

Breathwork techniques are particularly valuable for managing anxiety, including generalized anxiety disorder, social anxiety, and panic attacks. The act of focusing on one's breath can serve as a grounding and centering practice during moments of heightened anxiety. Techniques such as box breathing or 4-7-8 breathing provide a structured approach to calming the mind and alleviating anxious thoughts.

Emotional Regulation:

Breathwork can also aid in emotional regulation, helping individuals navigate their feelings more effectively. Mindful breathing practices encourage individuals to acknowledge and observe their emotions without judgment. This awareness allows for better emotional control and the ability to respond to situations with greater clarity and equanimity.

Improved Concentration and Mental Clarity:

Conscious breath control can enhance concentration and mental clarity. When individuals are mindful of their breathing patterns, they become more present in the moment and less prone to distractions. This heightened focus can improve cognitive performance, problem-solving abilities, and decision-making skills.

Enhanced Self-awareness:

Breathwork promotes self-awareness by encouraging individuals to connect with their inner experiences. As individuals become more attuned to their breath, they may gain insights into their thoughts, emotions, and bodily sensations. This self-awareness can be a powerful tool for personal growth and self-improvement.

Emotional Release and Healing:

Certain breathwork practices, such as Holotropic Breathwork, emphasize emotional release and healing. These techniques involve intense, intentional breathing patterns that can bring up suppressed emotions and memories. While the process can be challenging, it often leads to a sense of emotional catharsis and healing.

Mind-Body Connection:

Breathwork strengthens the mind-body connection by highlighting the interplay between physical sensations and emotional states. Individuals learn to recognize how changes in their breathing patterns correlate with shifts in their emotional well-being. This heightened awareness fosters a deeper understanding of the mind-body connection and how it impacts overall mental and emotional health.

Positive Mood Enhancement:

Breathwork can elevate one's mood and overall sense of well-being. Practices like Kapalabhati, which involve rapid and forceful exhalations followed by passive inhalations, are known to boost energy levels and create a sense of euphoria. Such techniques are often integrated into yoga and meditation practices to enhance positivity and vitality.

In conclusion, breathwork is a versatile and accessible practice that offers numerous benefits for mental and emotional well-being. By harnessing the power of conscious breathing, individuals can reduce stress, manage anxiety, improve emotional regulation, enhance concentration, and foster self-awareness. Whether through structured techniques or simply by cultivating mindful breathing habits, individuals have the opportunity to tap into the transformative potential of breathwork. As an integral component of holistic

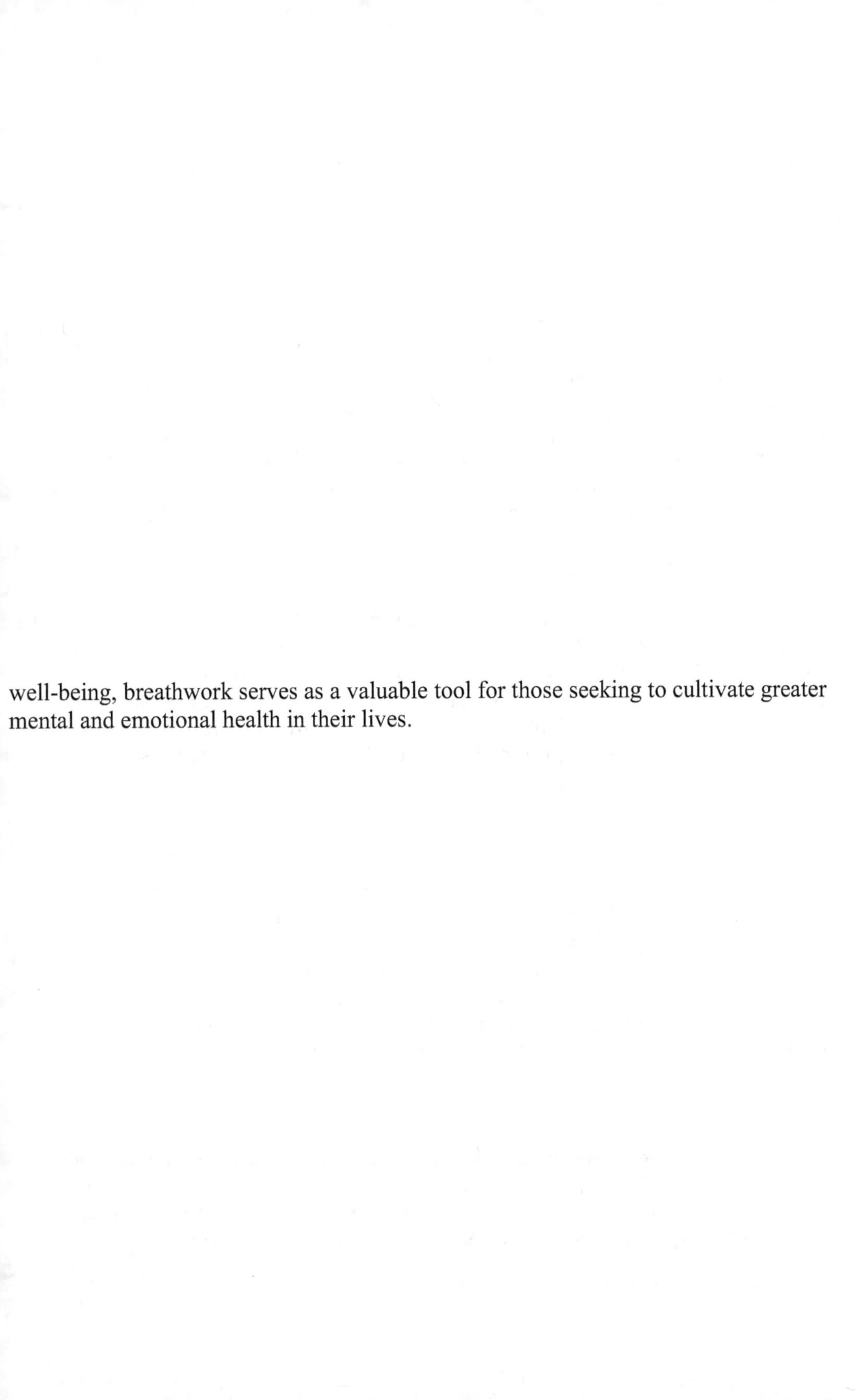

well-being, breathwork serves as a valuable tool for those seeking to cultivate greater mental and emotional health in their lives.

Integrating Breathwork with Other Holistic Practices

Integrating Breathwork with Other Holistic Practices

In the pursuit of holistic well-being, individuals often explore a variety of practices and techniques to nourish their mind, body, and spirit. One such practice that has shown remarkable synergy with other holistic approaches is breathwork. When integrated with complementary practices, breathwork becomes a powerful tool for enhancing overall wellness. In this essay, we will explore how breathwork can be harmoniously combined with other holistic practices to create a comprehensive approach to well-being.

Yoga and Breathwork:

Yoga and breathwork share a deep-rooted connection, making them a natural pairing. The practice of yoga involves physical postures (asanas), meditation, and breath control (pranayama). Pranayama, a fundamental aspect of yoga, focuses on conscious breathing techniques. When combined with yoga postures, pranayama enhances the mind-body connection, promotes relaxation, and deepens the meditative experience. Yogic breathing techniques such as Ujjayi and Bhastrika are often integrated into yoga classes to optimize the benefits of both practices.

Meditation and Breathwork:

Meditation and breathwork are complementary practices that amplify each other's effects. Meditation encourages mindfulness and the observation of thoughts and emotions without attachment. Breathwork serves as a gateway to mindfulness, providing individuals with a tangible point of focus—the breath. By using breathwork as a meditation anchor, individuals can achieve a state of deep relaxation and heightened awareness more readily. Techniques like mindfulness meditation often incorporate conscious breathing as a means of grounding and centering the practitioner.

Massage and Breathwork:

Massage therapy and breathwork form a holistic tandem for relaxation and stress relief. During a massage, the body's muscles and tissues are manipulated to release tension and promote circulation. Integrating conscious breathing into a massage session enhances the relaxation response. By focusing on their breath, individuals can let go of physical and emotional tension more effectively. Massage therapists may encourage clients to breathe deeply and mindfully during the session, resulting in a more profound sense of relaxation and well-being.

Aromatherapy and Breathwork:

Aromatherapy, which involves the use of essential oils to promote physical and emotional healing, pairs harmoniously with breathwork. Certain essential oils, such as lavender and eucalyptus, are known for their calming and respiratory benefits. Incorporating aromatherapy into a breathwork practice can enhance its effects. Individuals can inhale the soothing scents of essential oils while practicing breathwork, promoting relaxation and emotional balance.

Holistic Wellness Retreats:

Holistic wellness retreats often combine various practices, including yoga, meditation, massage, and breathwork, to create immersive and transformative experiences. Participants engage in a holistic approach to well-being, allowing them to explore and integrate these practices in a supportive environment. These retreats provide a structured and immersive way to experience the synergistic benefits of breathwork and other holistic techniques.

Tai Chi and Breathwork:

Tai Chi, an ancient Chinese martial art known for its graceful movements and meditation in motion, aligns well with breathwork. The slow, flowing movements of Tai Chi are synchronized with deep and intentional breathing. This combination fosters relaxation, balance, and improved energy flow (Qi or Chi). Tai Chi practitioners often emphasize diaphragmatic breathing, which supports overall health and vitality.

In conclusion, breathwork seamlessly integrates with various holistic practices, enriching their impact on overall well-being. Whether combined with yoga, meditation, massage, aromatherapy, or other holistic modalities, breathwork serves as a bridge to deeper self-awareness, relaxation, and vitality. These integrative approaches offer individuals a holistic toolkit for nurturing their physical, emotional, and spiritual dimensions. By embracing the interconnectedness of these practices, individuals can embark on a transformative journey toward greater well-being and harmony.

Specialized Breathwork Applications

Specialized Breathwork Applications

Breathwork, a practice focused on conscious control and regulation of breathing, offers a versatile set of techniques that can be tailored to address various physical, mental, and emotional needs. Beyond its general applications for stress reduction and relaxation, breathwork can be specialized to target specific issues or conditions. In this essay, we will explore some of the specialized applications of breathwork and how it can be harnessed to address unique challenges.

Breathwork for Anxiety and Panic Disorders:

Anxiety and panic disorders can be debilitating, but breathwork techniques can provide effective relief. One specialized approach is the 4-7-8 breathing method, which involves inhaling for four counts, holding for seven, and exhaling for eight. This technique activates the body's relaxation response, calming the nervous system and reducing anxiety levels. Practicing this breathwork regularly can help individuals manage their anxiety and panic attacks.

Breathwork for Sleep Disorders:

Many people struggle with sleep disorders, such as insomnia or sleep apnea. Specialized breathwork techniques can promote better sleep quality. The "4-7-8" technique mentioned earlier can be adapted for sleep by slowing the counts and focusing on deep, rhythmic breathing. Additionally, yoga-inspired breathing exercises like Nadi Shodhana (alternate nostril breathing) can relax the mind and prepare the body for restful sleep.

Breathwork for Pain Management:

Chronic pain conditions can significantly impact one's quality of life. Breathwork can be used as an adjunct to pain management strategies. Deep, diaphragmatic breathing can increase oxygenation, reduce muscle tension, and distract from the perception of pain. Visualization techniques, combined with breathwork, allow individuals to focus their attention away from discomfort, providing relief.

Breathwork for Athletic Performance:

Athletes can benefit from specialized breathwork to optimize their performance. Techniques like rhythmic breathing synchronization with physical exertion can improve endurance and maximize oxygen utilization. Controlled breath patterns can also help athletes stay focused, calm, and mentally resilient during competitions.

Breathwork for Trauma Recovery:

Individuals who have experienced trauma can find healing through specialized breathwork practices. Trauma-informed breathwork focuses on creating a safe environment for individuals to reconnect with their bodies and release stored emotional tension. Techniques like Somatic Experiencing, which incorporates breathwork, help survivors process and integrate traumatic experiences.

Breathwork for Respiratory Conditions:

For individuals with respiratory conditions like asthma or COPD, breathwork can be a valuable therapeutic tool. Pursed-lip breathing, for instance, involves inhaling through the nose and exhaling slowly through pursed lips. This technique helps maintain airway patency, reduce breathlessness, and improve oxygen exchange.

Breathwork for Emotional Release:

Breathwork can facilitate the release of stored emotions and trauma. Holotropic Breathwork, a specialized form of breathwork developed by Dr. Stanislav Grof, involves deep and rapid breathing to access altered states of consciousness. This process can lead to emotional catharsis and spiritual insights, promoting emotional healing and personal growth.

Breathwork for Cognitive Enhancement:

Some breathwork techniques are designed to enhance cognitive functions and mental clarity. The Kapalabhati technique, for instance, involves rapid and forceful exhalations followed by passive inhalations. This energizing breathwork can sharpen mental focus and invigorate the mind.

In conclusion, breathwork is a versatile practice with a wide range of specialized applications. From addressing anxiety and sleep disorders to enhancing athletic performance and aiding in trauma recovery, breathwork can be tailored to meet specific needs. When practiced under the guidance of a qualified instructor or therapist, specialized breathwork techniques have the potential to bring about transformative changes in physical, mental, and emotional well-being. As more research explores the efficacy of these specialized applications, breathwork continues to evolve as a valuable tool for holistic health and self-improvement.

Breathwork for Athletic Performance

Breathwork for Athletic Performance

Athletic performance is not only about physical strength and endurance but also about optimizing the body's capabilities to achieve peak results. One often-overlooked aspect of athletic performance is the breath, a fundamental physiological function that can be harnessed through breathwork techniques to enhance an athlete's performance. In this essay, we will explore how breathwork can play a vital role in improving athletic performance.

Improved Oxygen Utilization:

One of the primary benefits of breathwork for athletic performance is improved oxygen utilization. During strenuous physical activity, the body requires more oxygen to fuel muscles and energy production. Controlled and rhythmic breathing techniques can help ensure that the body receives a steady supply of oxygen. This can delay the onset of fatigue, allowing athletes to perform at a higher intensity for longer durations.

Enhancing Endurance:

Endurance athletes, such as long-distance runners and cyclists, can particularly benefit from breathwork. Techniques like "paced breathing" involve synchronizing breath with each step or pedal stroke. This rhythmic coordination helps maintain a consistent pace and prevents overexertion. It also helps athletes conserve energy, enabling them to endure longer and cover greater distances.

Managing Stress and Anxiety:

Competitive sports often come with a high level of stress and anxiety. Athletes who learn to control their breath can effectively manage these psychological factors. Deep and diaphragmatic breathing triggers the body's relaxation response, reducing stress hormone levels. This not only promotes better focus and concentration but also prevents the performance-diminishing effects of anxiety.

Mental Resilience:

Breathwork also enhances mental resilience, a critical factor in athletic success. Techniques like box breathing, which involves inhaling, holding, exhaling, and holding for equal counts, can help athletes stay composed under pressure. This controlled breathing calms the mind and reduces pre-competition jitters, allowing athletes to perform at their best.

Recovery and Injury Prevention:

Breathwork can expedite post-workout recovery and reduce the risk of injury. After intense exercise, controlled breathing helps remove excess carbon dioxide and metabolic waste from muscles, reducing soreness and inflammation. Additionally, breath-focused exercises, such as dynamic stretching with breath synchronization, can improve flexibility and reduce the likelihood of muscle strains.

Focusing the Mind:

A clear and focused mind is crucial in athletics. Breathwork techniques, such as mindfulness meditation with breath awareness, can sharpen an athlete's mental acuity. By training the mind to stay present and attentive, athletes can make quicker decisions, react more effectively to changing conditions, and stay in the zone during competitions.

Core Activation:

Proper breath control can also enhance core stability. Techniques like the "hollowing" breath engage the diaphragm and deep core muscles, providing a solid foundation for athletic movements. A strong core is essential for balance, power generation, and injury prevention.

Enhancing Recovery Breathing:

After a vigorous workout or competition, athletes can use breathwork to aid in recovery. Techniques like the 3:6:9 method, which involves inhaling for three counts, holding for six, and exhaling for nine, promote relaxation and recovery. This type of controlled exhalation helps return the body to a state of equilibrium.

In conclusion, breathwork is a valuable tool for enhancing athletic performance. Athletes who incorporate breathwork techniques into their training routines can experience improvements in endurance, stress management, mental resilience, and overall physical well-being. These techniques can be tailored to suit various sports and individual needs, making breathwork a versatile and accessible tool for athletes of all levels. As the awareness of breathwork's benefits continues to grow in the world of sports, it is likely to become an integral part of athletic training and performance optimization.

Breathwork in Clinical Settings

Breathwork in Clinical Settings

Breathwork, a collection of techniques aimed at controlling and optimizing one's breath, has gained recognition in clinical settings for its potential therapeutic benefits. This holistic approach to healing focuses on the mind-body connection, making it a valuable complement to traditional medical interventions. In this essay, we will explore the application of breathwork in clinical settings and its positive impact on physical and mental health.

Stress Reduction:

One of the primary applications of breathwork in clinical settings is stress reduction. Chronic stress has been linked to numerous health issues, including heart disease, depression, and anxiety disorders. Controlled breathing exercises, such as diaphragmatic breathing and deep breathing, can activate the body's relaxation response. This helps reduce stress hormone levels and promotes a sense of calm and well-being.

Anxiety and Panic Disorders:

Breathwork techniques are particularly effective in treating anxiety and panic disorders. Individuals suffering from these conditions often experience rapid, shallow breathing, which can exacerbate symptoms. Breathwork interventions teach patients to regain control of their breath, allowing them to manage and mitigate panic attacks. Techniques like box breathing, where one inhales, holds, exhales, and holds for equal counts, are especially useful in these situations.

PTSD and Trauma Recovery:

Post-Traumatic Stress Disorder (PTSD) and trauma survivors can benefit significantly from breathwork therapies. Traumatic experiences often lead to hypervigilance and emotional dysregulation. Breathwork helps individuals release trapped emotional energy and promotes a sense of safety and grounding. This can be instrumental in trauma recovery, providing a foundation for further therapeutic work.

Pain Management:

Chronic pain conditions, such as fibromyalgia and chronic back pain, can be debilitating. Breathwork can be incorporated into pain management strategies to reduce the perception of pain. By focusing on slow, deep breaths and mindfulness, patients can redirect their attention away from pain, resulting in increased comfort and improved quality of life.

Respiratory Conditions:

Breathwork is also valuable for individuals with respiratory conditions, such as asthma and chronic obstructive pulmonary disease (COPD). Breathing exercises like pursed-lip breathing and the Buteyko method can improve lung function and oxygen utilization. These techniques help patients breathe more efficiently, reduce breathlessness, and enhance their overall respiratory health.

Sleep Disorders:

Many individuals suffer from sleep disorders like insomnia and sleep apnea. Irregular breathing patterns are often associated with these conditions. Breathwork practices, such as progressive muscle relaxation with breath synchronization, can induce relaxation and improve sleep quality by regulating breathing patterns and reducing nighttime awakenings.

Mood Disorders:

Breathwork can be an adjunctive therapy for mood disorders like depression and bipolar disorder. The deep breathing and mindfulness aspects of breathwork can help stabilize mood and alleviate symptoms of sadness and emotional instability. Regular practice can enhance emotional resilience and well-being.

Enhanced Emotional Awareness:

Breathwork encourages individuals to become more attuned to their emotional states. As patients learn to observe their breath and its connection to their emotions, they gain insight into their mental and physical well-being. This heightened self-awareness can lead to better emotional regulation and greater emotional intelligence.

In conclusion, breathwork is a versatile and valuable therapeutic tool in clinical settings. Its ability to address stress, anxiety, trauma, pain, respiratory conditions, sleep disorders, and mood disorders makes it a holistic approach to improving overall health and well-being. As the field of integrative medicine continues to expand, breathwork is gaining recognition as an effective and accessible modality for enhancing patient outcomes. It empowers individuals to take an active role in their healing process, promoting a sense of agency and self-efficacy. With ongoing research and the integration of breathwork into

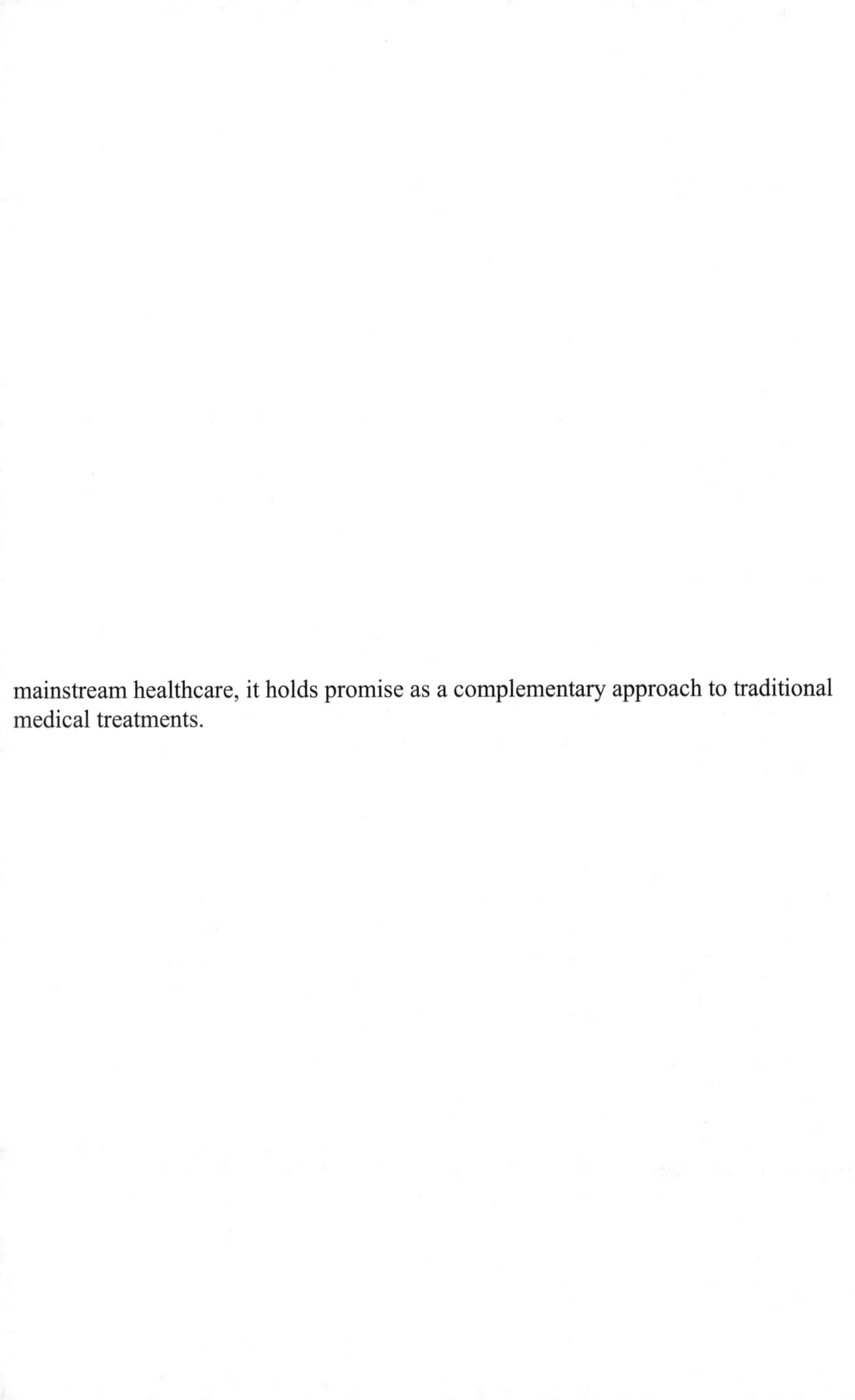

mainstream healthcare, it holds promise as a complementary approach to traditional medical treatments.

Breathwork for Personal Growth and Transformation

Breathwork for Personal Growth and Transformation

Breathwork, a practice centered around conscious control and manipulation of one's breath, has emerged as a powerful tool for personal growth and transformation. While it has ancient roots in various spiritual and healing traditions, modern breathwork techniques have gained popularity for their potential to facilitate profound changes in individuals' lives. In this essay, we will explore how breathwork can be harnessed for personal growth and transformation.

Self-Awareness and Mindfulness:

At the core of breathwork is the practice of becoming acutely aware of one's breath. This heightened awareness naturally extends to one's thoughts, emotions, and bodily sensations. Through mindful breathing, individuals gain insight into their mental and emotional states, paving the way for self-discovery and self-awareness. This process of introspection is essential for personal growth, as it allows individuals to recognize patterns, triggers, and areas of improvement.

Stress Reduction and Relaxation:

Breathwork techniques are highly effective in reducing stress and promoting relaxation. By engaging in deep, controlled breathing, individuals activate the body's parasympathetic nervous system, which counteracts the stress response. This results in lowered stress hormone levels, reduced muscle tension, and an overall sense of calm. As stress is a significant obstacle to personal growth, breathwork provides a foundation for emotional resilience and personal development.

Emotional Release and Healing:

Many individuals carry emotional baggage from past experiences, which can hinder personal growth. Breathwork can act as a catalyst for emotional release and healing. Through techniques like "cathartic breathwork," individuals can access and release suppressed emotions. This process can be transformative, as it allows individuals to let go of emotional burdens, enabling personal growth and self-empowerment.

Overcoming Fears and Limiting Beliefs:

Breathwork can help individuals confront and overcome their fears and limiting beliefs. By deliberately altering their breathing patterns, individuals can enter altered states of consciousness that allow for deep exploration of their psyche. This altered state can facilitate the examination of subconscious thought patterns and beliefs, enabling individuals to challenge and reframe them. This process empowers individuals to break free from self-imposed limitations and fosters personal growth.

Enhancing Creativity and Intuition:

Breathwork has been associated with enhanced creativity and intuition. Through focused breathwork sessions, individuals can tap into their creative potential and gain access to their inner wisdom. The state of heightened awareness achieved through breathwork can lead to insights, innovations, and a deeper connection to one's intuition, all of which contribute to personal growth and self-actualization.

Improved Mental Clarity and Focus:

Breathwork practices can improve mental clarity and focus. Deep and rhythmic breathing oxygenates the brain, enhancing cognitive function and concentration. This heightened mental clarity can be harnessed to set and achieve personal growth goals with greater precision and effectiveness.

Spiritual Exploration and Connection:

For those on a spiritual journey, breathwork can facilitate profound spiritual experiences and connections. Certain breathwork techniques, such as holotropic breathwork, can induce altered states of consciousness, leading to mystical or transcendent experiences. These experiences can provide a deeper sense of purpose and interconnectedness, contributing to personal growth and transformation.

Integrating Body, Mind, and Spirit:

Breathwork integrates the body, mind, and spirit into a holistic experience. It fosters a sense of unity and balance among these aspects of self. This integration is fundamental to personal growth, as it aligns one's actions, thoughts, and emotions with their authentic self.

In conclusion, breathwork is a versatile and potent tool for personal growth and transformation. It offers a pathway to self-awareness, emotional release, overcoming limitations, enhancing creativity, improving mental clarity, and connecting with one's spiritual self. As individuals embark on their personal growth journeys, breathwork can serve as a valuable companion, helping them navigate challenges and realize their full potential. With its myriad of benefits, breathwork continues to gain recognition as a holistic practice that empowers individuals to achieve profound and lasting personal transformation.

The Practice of Breathwork

The Practice of Breathwork

Breathwork is an ancient practice that has gained significant attention in recent years for its myriad of physical, mental, and emotional benefits. Rooted in various cultures and traditions, breathwork involves conscious control and manipulation of the breath to achieve specific outcomes. In this essay, we will explore the practice of breathwork, its historical origins, and its modern applications.

Historical Origins:

Breathwork is not a new phenomenon; its roots can be traced back thousands of years. Various cultures and spiritual traditions recognized the profound connection between breath and well-being. For example, in yoga, the term "pranayama" refers to breath control techniques that have been practiced for centuries. Ancient Chinese, Greek, and Egyptian cultures also incorporated breathwork into their healing and spiritual practices.

Basic Principles:

At its core, breathwork revolves around the fundamental principle that the breath is a bridge between the body and mind. It involves deliberate manipulation of the breath to influence physical, mental, and emotional states. The practice can be as simple as deep, slow breathing or as complex as specific techniques designed to achieve particular outcomes.

Breathwork Techniques:

Breathwork encompasses a wide range of techniques, each with its unique purpose and approach. Some of the most commonly practiced techniques include:

Diaphragmatic Breathing: This technique focuses on deep abdominal breathing, engaging the diaphragm to expand the lungs fully. It promotes relaxation and oxygenates the body.

Box Breathing: Box breathing involves inhaling, holding, exhaling, and holding the breath in equal intervals. It can help reduce stress and improve focus.

Circular Breathing: Commonly used in playing wind instruments, circular breathing involves a continuous cycle of inhaling through the nose and exhaling through the mouth, allowing for uninterrupted airflow.

Holotropic Breathwork: Developed by Dr. Stanislav Grof, this technique involves rapid and deep breathing to induce altered states of consciousness, facilitating emotional release and spiritual experiences.

Buteyko Breathing: Designed to address breathing disorders, this technique focuses on shallow breathing and reducing excessive breathing to improve overall health.

Modern Applications:

In contemporary society, breathwork has found applications in various fields, including:

Stress Reduction: The practice of breathwork is well-known for its stress-reducing benefits. By engaging the parasympathetic nervous system, controlled breathing can lower stress hormone levels and induce a state of relaxation.

Mental Clarity and Focus: Deep, rhythmic breathing oxygenates the brain, improving cognitive function and concentration. This makes breathwork a valuable tool for enhancing mental clarity and focus.

Emotional Regulation: Breathwork techniques can help individuals manage and regulate their emotions. By consciously altering their breath, individuals can modulate their emotional responses and achieve a greater sense of emotional balance.

Physical Health: Breathwork can be used to improve physical health by increasing lung capacity, enhancing oxygen uptake, and promoting overall cardiovascular well-being.

Spiritual Growth: Many individuals use breathwork as a means of spiritual exploration and growth. Techniques like holotropic breathwork and circular breathing can induce altered states of consciousness that lead to profound spiritual experiences.

Conclusion:

Breathwork is a versatile and accessible practice with deep historical roots and modern applications. Whether used for stress reduction, mental clarity, emotional regulation, physical health, or spiritual growth, breathwork offers a holistic approach to well-being. As more individuals recognize the power of their breath, the practice of breathwork continues to evolve and adapt to meet the needs of a modern world seeking balance, health, and self-awareness.

Developing a Personal Breathwork Practice

Developing a Personal Breathwork Practice

Breathwork is a powerful practice that can bring about numerous physical, mental, and emotional benefits. Whether you're looking to reduce stress, enhance mental clarity, or improve your overall well-being, developing a personal breathwork practice can be a transformative journey. In this essay, we will explore the steps to develop your own breathwork practice.

Step Education and Understanding

Before embarking on your breathwork journey, it's essential to educate yourself about the different techniques and approaches available. There are various schools of thought and methods, such as diaphragmatic breathing, box breathing, and holotropic breathwork, each with its unique principles and objectives. Take the time to research and understand these techniques, as well as their potential benefits and contraindications.

Step Setting Clear Intentions

Once you have a basic understanding of breathwork, it's crucial to set clear intentions for your practice. What do you hope to achieve through breathwork? Are you looking to reduce stress, improve focus, or explore your inner self? Having specific intentions will guide your practice and help you choose the most suitable techniques.

Step Finding a Suitable Space

Creating a conducive environment for your breathwork practice is essential. Find a quiet, comfortable space where you won't be disturbed. It could be a corner of your home, a peaceful outdoor setting, or a dedicated meditation area. Ensuring that your practice space is free from distractions can enhance your experience.

Step Consistency and Routine

Consistency is key to reaping the benefits of breathwork. Establish a routine that works for you, whether it's a daily practice or several times a week. Setting aside dedicated time for your breathwork sessions will help you integrate the practice into your life more effectively.

Step Start with the Basics

For beginners, it's advisable to start with basic breathwork techniques. Diaphragmatic breathing, for example, is a foundational practice that involves deep abdominal breathing. It's an excellent starting point for building awareness of your breath and its effects on your body and mind.

Step Explore and Experiment

As you become more comfortable with your practice, don't hesitate to explore and experiment with different breathwork techniques. Try out techniques like box breathing or circular breathing to see how they resonate with you. Keep an open mind and be willing to adapt your practice based on your experiences.

Step Guided Sessions and Teachers

Consider seeking guidance from experienced breathwork practitioners or teachers, especially if you're new to the practice. Guided sessions can provide valuable insights, help you refine your technique, and ensure that you're practicing safely. Many skilled instructors offer workshops, classes, or online resources to support your journey.

Step Self-Reflection and Journaling

Maintaining a breathwork journal can be a valuable tool for self-reflection. After each session, take a few moments to jot down your experiences, thoughts, and emotions. Over time, this journal can help you track your progress, identify patterns, and gain deeper insights into the impact of your practice.

Step Trust the Process

Breathwork is a personal journey, and it's essential to trust the process. Your experiences may vary from session to session, and that's perfectly normal. Allow yourself to surrender to the practice without judgment or expectations. Trust that your breath will guide you toward the healing and growth you seek.

Step 10: Integration into Daily Life

Finally, aim to integrate the principles of breathwork into your daily life. As you become more attuned to your breath, you can use its power to remain centered and mindful throughout your day. Simple practices like taking a few deep breaths during moments of stress or tension can have a profound impact on your overall well-being.

In conclusion, developing a personal breathwork practice is a journey of self-discovery and transformation. By educating yourself, setting intentions, creating a suitable environment, and maintaining consistency, you can harness the power of your breath to enhance your physical, mental, and emotional health. Whether you're a beginner or an experienced practitioner, breathwork offers a path to greater self-awareness, balance, and inner peace.

Challenges and Tips for Effective Practice

Challenges and Tips for Effective Practice

Breathwork is a transformative practice that offers numerous benefits, from stress reduction to enhanced mental clarity. However, like any endeavor, it comes with its challenges. In this essay, we will explore some common challenges faced during breathwork practice and provide tips for overcoming them.

Challenge Restlessness and Distraction

One of the most common challenges during breathwork is dealing with restlessness and distraction. It's natural for the mind to wander and for external distractions to arise, especially in the early stages of practice.

Tip: To address this challenge, start with short practice sessions and gradually extend the duration as you build your concentration. Additionally, using techniques like mindfulness meditation or listening to calming music can help anchor your focus during breathwork.

Challenge Breath Awareness

Maintaining awareness of your breath, especially during busy or stressful times, can be challenging. It's easy to slip into shallow breathing or forget to practice altogether.

Tip: To enhance breath awareness, set regular reminders on your phone or create cues in your environment to prompt you to take a few mindful breaths throughout the day. This will help you integrate breathwork into your daily routine.

Challenge Overthinking

Overthinking, analyzing, or expecting specific outcomes from your breathwork practice can hinder its effectiveness. The desire for immediate results can create unnecessary pressure.

Tip: Let go of expectations and simply allow your breath to flow naturally. Trust the process and focus on the present moment. Remember that the benefits of breathwork may become more apparent with consistent practice over time.

Challenge Physical Discomfort

Physical discomfort, such as stiffness, discomfort in certain postures, or tension, can detract from the experience of breathwork.

Tip: Ensure you practice breathwork in a comfortable and supportive environment. Use props like pillows or bolsters to enhance comfort during seated or lying positions. If you experience discomfort, adjust your posture or explore alternative positions to find what works best for you.

Challenge Impatience

Impatience can be a significant challenge, especially for those seeking immediate relief from stress or emotional turmoil. Breathwork is a gradual process, and its benefits may not be instantly apparent.

Tip: Practice patience and perseverance. Understand that breathwork is a journey, and its effects may unfold over time. Celebrate small victories and acknowledge the incremental changes in your well-being.

Challenge Lack of Consistency

Inconsistent practice can limit the effectiveness of breathwork. Life's demands and busy schedules can make it challenging to prioritize daily practice.

Tip: Establish a consistent routine that suits your lifestyle. Even short daily sessions can yield significant benefits. Treat your breathwork practice as an essential self-care ritual, and it will become easier to maintain.

Challenge Self-Judgment

Self-judgment and self-criticism can surface during breathwork, especially when challenging emotions or thoughts arise.

Tip: Cultivate self-compassion and non-judgmental awareness. Understand that breathwork provides a safe space for exploring your inner world, and there are no right or wrong experiences. Embrace whatever arises with curiosity and kindness.

Challenge Seeking Guidance

Many individuals seek guidance during their breathwork practice, whether through workshops, classes, or with a trained instructor. Finding the right guidance can be a challenge.

Tip: Research and explore different sources of guidance. Attend workshops or classes led by experienced instructors who resonate with you. Online resources, books, and apps can also provide valuable guidance and support for your practice.

In conclusion, while breathwork offers numerous benefits for physical, mental, and emotional well-being, it's essential to recognize and address the challenges that may arise during your practice. By acknowledging and implementing these tips, you can navigate and overcome common obstacles, allowing your breathwork practice to flourish. Remember that breathwork is a personal journey, and with patience, consistency, and self-compassion, you can unlock its full potential for healing and transformation.

Measuring Progress and Outcomes

Measuring Progress and Outcomes in Breathwork

Breathwork is a powerful practice that can lead to a range of physical, mental, and emotional benefits. While these benefits are often subjective and personal, it is essential to find ways to measure progress and outcomes to understand the impact of your breathwork practice. In this essay, we will explore various methods for measuring progress and outcomes in breathwork.

Self-Reflection and Journaling

One of the most accessible and effective ways to measure progress in breathwork is through self-reflection and journaling. By keeping a record of your experiences, thoughts, and emotions before and after each session, you can track changes over time.

How to Do It: Set aside a few minutes before and after your breathwork practice to jot down your feelings, thoughts, and any notable sensations. Over time, review your journal entries to identify patterns, shifts in mood, or changes in your overall well-being.

Breath Awareness and Control

An immediate and tangible outcome of regular breathwork practice is improved breath awareness and control. Measuring your breath patterns and capacities can provide valuable insights into your progress.

How to Do It: Use a simple breath monitoring tool, such as a spirometer or a smartphone app designed for tracking breath rate and depth. Record your baseline measurements and periodically check to see if there are any improvements.

Stress Reduction and Relaxation

Many people turn to breathwork to reduce stress and induce relaxation. Assessing your stress levels and relaxation can help gauge the effectiveness of your practice.

How to Do It: Consider using stress assessment scales or biofeedback devices to measure physiological markers like heart rate variability (HRV) before and after breathwork sessions. Decreased stress levels and increased HRV are indicative of progress.

Improved Sleep Patterns

Breathwork can positively impact sleep quality and patterns. Monitoring your sleep can provide valuable data on the impact of your practice.

How to Do It: Use a sleep tracking device or smartphone app to record your sleep duration, quality, and disturbances. Pay attention to any improvements in your sleep patterns, such as falling asleep faster or waking up more refreshed.

Emotional Well-being

Emotional well-being is a significant outcome of breathwork. Measuring your emotional state can help you understand the impact of the practice on your mood and emotional resilience.

How to Do It: Use mood tracking apps or self-assessment questionnaires to measure your emotional state regularly. Look for changes in mood, such as reduced anxiety, increased feelings of calmness, or improved emotional regulation.

Physical Health Metrics

For those seeking physical health benefits from breathwork, tracking relevant health metrics can be essential. These may include blood pressure, heart rate, and lung function.

How to Do It: Regularly measure your blood pressure and heart rate before and after breathwork sessions to monitor any changes. If you have specific health conditions, consult with a healthcare professional to establish relevant baseline metrics and track progress.

Performance Enhancement

If you are using breathwork to improve athletic or physical performance, measuring performance metrics is crucial.

How to Do It: Keep records of your athletic or physical achievements, such as running times, strength gains, or endurance levels. Assess whether your breathwork practice has contributed to improved performance.

Psychological Assessments

Psychological assessments and tests can provide valuable insights into your mental well-being and cognitive functioning.

How to Do It: Take psychological assessments or cognitive tests before and after an extended period of breathwork practice. Look for changes in cognitive functioning, memory, and emotional resilience.

Feedback from Others

Sometimes, it can be challenging to gauge your progress on your own. Seek feedback from friends, family, or a therapist who can provide an external perspective on changes they've observed.

How to Do It: Ask trusted individuals for their observations regarding your mood, behavior, and overall well-being. Their input can offer valuable insights.

In conclusion, measuring progress and outcomes in breathwork is essential for understanding the impact of this transformative practice. Whether through self-reflection, monitoring physical health metrics, or seeking feedback from others, there are various methods to assess the benefits of breathwork. By using these measurement techniques, you can gain a deeper understanding of how breathwork positively influences your life and well-being. Remember that progress may be gradual, and consistent practice is key to realizing the full potential of breathwork in your life.

Breathwork in Different Cultures and Traditions

Breathwork in Different Cultures and Traditions

Breathwork, the practice of consciously controlling one's breath, is a powerful tool for self-improvement and well-being that has been embraced by various cultures and traditions throughout history. While the specific techniques and philosophies may differ, the fundamental understanding of the breath's significance remains a common thread. In this essay, we will explore the diverse ways in which breathwork is incorporated into different cultures and traditions.

Yoga and Pranayama in India

One of the most well-known practices of breathwork is pranayama, a vital component of yoga in India. Pranayama involves breath control techniques aimed at harnessing life force energy, or prana, within the body. It is considered an essential step towards spiritual growth and self-realization in Indian traditions.

Qigong and Daoism in China

China has a rich history of breathwork practices, particularly in the context of Qigong and Daoism. Qigong involves a combination of breath control, meditation, and movement to cultivate and balance the body's vital energy, known as "qi" or "chi." Daoist philosophy emphasizes the harmonization of the body's energies, and breathwork plays a pivotal role in achieving this balance.

Holotropic Breathwork in the West

Holotropic Breathwork, developed by psychiatrist Stanislav Grof, is a form of breathwork that gained popularity in the West. It combines deep and rhythmic breathing with evocative music to facilitate altered states of consciousness and self-exploration. This approach is often used for personal growth, healing, and psychotherapy.

Indigenous Practices and Shamanism

Many indigenous cultures around the world incorporate breathwork into their spiritual and healing practices. Shamans, or spiritual leaders, often use breathwork techniques to induce altered states of consciousness, connect with the spirit world, and facilitate healing. These practices vary widely across different indigenous traditions.

Sufism and Whirling Dervishes

Within the mystical tradition of Sufism in Islam, the Sufis practice a unique form of breathwork during the "dhikr" or remembrance of God. This practice involves rhythmic breathing and chanting to attain a state of spiritual ecstasy. The famous Whirling Dervishes of the Mevlevi Order use spinning as a form of breathwork to achieve a profound connection with the divine.

Buddhist Meditation Techniques

Buddhism incorporates breathwork into various meditation techniques. Mindfulness of breath, or "anapanasati," is a foundational practice in Buddhist traditions. Practitioners focus on their breath to cultivate awareness, concentration, and insight, ultimately leading to enlightenment.

Native American Sweat Lodge Ceremonies

Native American tribes conduct sweat lodge ceremonies that include a breathwork element. Participants sit in a heated enclosure and engage in deep breathing exercises to purify their bodies, minds, and spirits. These ceremonies are often considered a form of spiritual rebirth.

Wim Hof Method

The Wim Hof Method, developed by "The Iceman" Wim Hof, combines specific breathwork techniques with cold exposure and meditation. This approach aims to enhance physical and mental performance, improve immunity, and increase overall well-being. It has gained popularity in recent years for its potential health benefits.

Christian Contemplative Prayer

In Christian contemplative traditions, breathwork is used as a means of deepening one's relationship with God. Practitioners often engage in rhythmic breathing and meditative prayer to achieve a state of communion with the divine.

In conclusion, breathwork is a universal practice that transcends cultural and geographical boundaries. It has been integrated into diverse cultures and traditions, each with its unique approach and purpose. Whether used for spiritual enlightenment, healing, personal growth, or physical well-being, breathwork continues to be a valuable tool for individuals seeking a deeper connection with themselves and the world around them. As we explore the global tapestry of breathwork traditions, we gain a greater appreciation for the profound impact of conscious breathing on the human experience.

Eastern Traditions of Breathwork

Eastern Traditions of Breathwork

Breathwork is a practice that has been central to Eastern traditions for thousands of years. These traditions recognize the profound connection between the breath, the mind, and the body, using breathwork as a means of achieving physical, mental, and spiritual well-being. In this essay, we will delve into some of the Eastern traditions of breathwork and their significance.

Pranayama in Yoga:

Perhaps the most well-known Eastern tradition of breathwork is pranayama, which plays a vital role in the practice of yoga. In Sanskrit, "prana" means life force, and "yama" means control or restraint. Pranayama involves various breathing techniques designed to control and harness prana for physical and spiritual benefits.

One of the most basic pranayama techniques is "Ujjayi" breathing, characterized by a soft hissing sound produced by slightly constricting the throat during inhalation and exhalation. This technique calms the mind, enhances concentration, and facilitates the flow of energy in the body.

Anapanasati in Buddhism:

Anapanasati, or mindfulness of breathing, is a fundamental practice in Buddhist meditation traditions. It involves focusing one's attention on the breath, observing it without attempting to control it. This practice cultivates mindfulness and concentration, essential qualities for insight and enlightenment in Buddhism.

Breathing meditation encourages practitioners to observe the breath as it naturally rises and falls, grounding them in the present moment and helping them develop a deeper understanding of the impermanent nature of reality.

Taoist Breathing in Daoism:

Daoist philosophy emphasizes harmony with the Tao, the fundamental principle that underlies everything in the universe. Breathwork, known as Daoist breathing, is a core practice in achieving this harmony. Daoist practitioners engage in gentle, deep abdominal breathing to align themselves with the natural rhythms of the universe.

Qi Gong Practices:

Qi Gong is a holistic system of coordinated body posture and movement, meditation, and breathwork. It aims to cultivate and balance the body's vital energy, known as "qi" or "chi." Qi Gong exercises often include specific breathwork techniques designed to enhance the flow of qi within the body.

One well-known Qi Gong practice is the "Eight Brocades," which involves a series of movements coordinated with deep and rhythmic breathing. This practice is believed to promote physical health, mental clarity, and longevity.

Sufi Breathing in Islam:

Within the mystical tradition of Sufism in Islam, Sufis use breathwork to achieve a state of spiritual ecstasy and union with the divine. Through rhythmic and intentional breathing, Sufis aim to transcend their physical limitations and connect with the spiritual realm.

The Sufi practice of "dhikr" involves chanting and deep breathing to reach altered states of consciousness. This practice is a means of remembrance and communion with God.

Traditional Chinese Medicine (TCM):

In Traditional Chinese Medicine, breathwork is considered a fundamental aspect of health and healing. TCM practitioners emphasize the balance and harmonization of the body's vital energies, known as "qi" and "jing." Breathwork techniques, such as "dao yin," focus on regulating and cultivating these energies for health and longevity.

In conclusion, Eastern traditions of breathwork have played a significant role in promoting physical, mental, and spiritual well-being for millennia. These practices emphasize the profound connection between the breath, the mind, and the body, offering valuable tools for self-awareness, health, and spiritual growth. As more people around the world recognize the benefits of Eastern breathwork traditions, the ancient wisdom of conscious breathing continues to enrich lives and promote holistic wellness.

Western Approaches to Breathwork

Western Approaches to Breathwork

While the practice of breathwork has ancient roots in Eastern traditions, it has also found its place in Western approaches to health and well-being. Over the years, Western practitioners and researchers have developed and embraced various breathwork techniques, recognizing their potential to enhance physical, mental, and emotional health. In this essay, we will explore some of the Western approaches to breathwork and their significance.

The Feldenkrais Method:

Developed by Israeli physicist and engineer Moshe Feldenkrais, the Feldenkrais Method is an educational approach that emphasizes self-awareness and improved movement. A fundamental aspect of this method is awareness of one's breath and its connection to movement and overall body function. Practitioners use gentle movements and breath awareness to release tension, improve posture, and promote relaxation.

The Buteyko Method:

The Buteyko Method, created by Russian doctor Konstantin Buteyko, focuses on retraining the breath to alleviate various health issues, particularly respiratory conditions such as asthma and allergies. This method emphasizes nasal breathing and reducing excessive breathing patterns, which can lead to a range of health problems. By adopting specific breathing exercises, practitioners aim to improve oxygen utilization and overall well-being.

Holotropic Breathwork:

Developed by psychiatrist Stanislav Grof and his wife Christina Grof, Holotropic Breathwork is a therapeutic practice that uses deep and controlled breathing to induce altered states of consciousness. Participants engage in extended breathwork sessions to explore their subconscious, release emotional trauma, and gain insights into their inner selves. Holotropic Breathwork has gained popularity in Western psychology and self-development circles as a means of promoting personal growth and healing.

Breathwork in Psychotherapy:

Several Western psychotherapists have integrated breathwork into their therapeutic practices to help clients address emotional and psychological issues. Breathwork in psychotherapy often involves guided breathing exercises that facilitate emotional release, stress reduction, and relaxation. It can be particularly effective in addressing trauma, anxiety, and depression.

Transformational Breathwork:

Transformational Breathwork, developed by Judith Kravitz, combines conscious breathing with various bodywork techniques to create a holistic approach to healing and self-improvement. Practitioners engage in specific breathing patterns aimed at expanding lung capacity and promoting emotional release. This method is used to address a wide range of physical, emotional, and spiritual issues.

Integrative Breathwork:

Integrative Breathwork, also known as Integrative Breathwork Therapy (IBT), combines elements of psychology, spirituality, and bodywork to facilitate healing and personal growth. This approach utilizes various breathing techniques to address issues such as trauma, stress, and addiction. By connecting the mind, body, and breath, individuals can gain insights into their patterns and make positive changes in their lives.

Breathwork for Stress Reduction:

In Western societies, where stress and anxiety are prevalent, many individuals turn to breathwork as a practical tool for managing these challenges. Techniques such as diaphragmatic breathing and mindful breathing are taught in therapeutic settings, workplaces, and wellness programs to help people reduce stress levels, improve focus, and enhance overall mental well-being.

In conclusion, Western approaches to breathwork have embraced and adapted ancient practices to meet the needs of contemporary society. From therapeutic applications to stress reduction and personal growth, breathwork has found a valuable place in Western health and wellness practices. These approaches emphasize the profound connection between breath, the mind, and the body, offering practical tools for individuals seeking to enhance their physical, mental, and emotional well-being. As more research and understanding of breathwork continue to develop in Western cultures, it is likely that these practices will continue to play a significant role in promoting holistic health and personal transformation.

Scientific Insights into Breathwork

Scientific Insights into Breathwork

Breathwork, often associated with ancient practices from Eastern traditions, has been gaining recognition in recent years for its potential to improve physical, mental, and emotional well-being. Beyond its historical and cultural roots, breathwork is now a subject of scientific inquiry, with researchers exploring its mechanisms and benefits. In this essay, we will delve into the scientific insights into breathwork and its impact on human health.

Breathwork and Stress Reduction:

One of the most extensively studied areas in breathwork is its role in stress reduction. Scientific investigations have shown that specific breathing techniques can activate the body's relaxation response, leading to decreased cortisol levels (the stress hormone) and improved overall mental well-being. Deep breathing exercises, such as diaphragmatic breathing and coherent breathing, have been found to help individuals manage stress more effectively.

Impact on the Autonomic Nervous System:

The autonomic nervous system (ANS) plays a crucial role in regulating bodily functions, including heart rate, blood pressure, and digestion. Breathwork has been found to influence the ANS, shifting it from a state of sympathetic dominance (fight-or-flight response) to parasympathetic dominance (rest and digest). This shift can lead to reduced stress, lower heart rate, and improved digestion.

Influence on Brain Function:

Research using neuroimaging techniques, such as functional magnetic resonance imaging (fMRI) and electroencephalography (EEG), has revealed that breathwork can have a profound impact on brain function. Specific breathing practices, like mindfulness meditation and pranayama, have been associated with increased activity in brain regions responsible for attention, emotional regulation, and memory. These findings suggest that breathwork can enhance cognitive functioning and emotional resilience.

Breathing and Emotional Regulation:

Emotions and breathing are closely interconnected. Scientific studies have shown that breathwork can influence emotional states by modulating brain areas responsible for emotional processing. Techniques like paced breathing and alternate nostril breathing have been associated with improved emotional regulation and mood enhancement. These findings highlight the potential of breathwork as a tool for managing conditions like anxiety and depression.

Respiratory Health and Lung Function:

Breathwork exercises that focus on improving breathing mechanics can have a positive impact on respiratory health. Research has demonstrated that practices like the Buteyko Method, which emphasizes nasal breathing and reduced breathing volume, can help individuals with asthma and other respiratory conditions. Additionally, deep breathing exercises can enhance lung capacity and oxygen exchange efficiency.

Cardiovascular Benefits:

Breathwork has shown promise in improving cardiovascular health. Studies have indicated that techniques such as slow and controlled breathing can lead to reduced blood pressure and improved heart rate variability, which is associated with better cardiovascular outcomes. These findings suggest that breathwork may be a complementary approach to managing hypertension and cardiovascular diseases.

Immune System Modulation:

Emerging research suggests that breathwork may influence the immune system. Deep breathing practices have been associated with increased levels of natural killer cells, which play a crucial role in the body's defense against infections and cancer. While more research is needed in this area, these initial findings indicate a potential link between breathwork and immune system modulation.

In conclusion, scientific insights into breathwork are shedding light on its mechanisms and potential benefits. From stress reduction and emotional regulation to improvements in respiratory health and cardiovascular function, research has provided compelling evidence for the positive impact of breathwork on human well-being. As our understanding of breathwork continues to evolve, it is likely that its therapeutic applications will expand, offering individuals valuable tools for enhancing their physical, mental, and emotional health. Breathwork is no longer solely a domain of ancient traditions; it is now a subject of scientific exploration that holds promise for improving the quality of life for many people.

Research on Breathing and Physiology

Research on Breathing and Physiology

Breathwork, the intentional practice of controlling one's breath, has garnered increasing attention from researchers interested in understanding its effects on human physiology. While the roots of breathwork lie in ancient traditions and cultures, modern science has begun to uncover the intricate relationship between breathing and the body's physiological responses. In this essay, we will explore the fascinating research on breathing and its impact on various aspects of human physiology.

Respiratory Rate and Oxygenation:

One of the fundamental aspects of breathwork research focuses on the respiratory rate and its influence on oxygenation. Studies have shown that slow, controlled breathing can enhance oxygen uptake and improve blood oxygen levels. For example, deep diaphragmatic breathing techniques, commonly practiced in yoga and mindfulness, have been associated with increased oxygen saturation in the bloodstream. This research highlights the importance of conscious breathing in optimizing the body's oxygen supply.

Heart Rate Variability (HRV):

Heart rate variability is a measure of the variation in time between successive heartbeats and is indicative of the autonomic nervous system's functioning. Research has demonstrated that specific breathwork techniques, such as coherent breathing, can lead to increased HRV. Higher HRV is associated with greater adaptability to stress, improved cardiovascular health, and enhanced overall well-being. These findings suggest that breathwork can play a crucial role in promoting a healthy heart and nervous system.

Blood Pressure Regulation:

Breathwork has been investigated for its potential to regulate blood pressure. Controlled breathing exercises, particularly those emphasizing slow exhalations, have been shown to lead to reductions in both systolic and diastolic blood pressure. These findings have significant implications for individuals with hypertension and cardiovascular conditions, offering a non-pharmacological approach to managing blood pressure.

Stress Response and Hormones:

The stress response is intricately linked to breathing patterns. Research has unveiled the connection between specific breathwork practices and the body's stress hormones, particularly cortisol. Deep, rhythmic breathing exercises have been associated with decreased cortisol levels, suggesting that breathwork can help mitigate the detrimental effects of chronic stress. Moreover, studies have indicated that regular breathwork may improve overall stress resilience.

Immune Function:

Emerging research has explored the relationship between breathwork and immune function. Some studies have suggested that certain breathing techniques, such as the Wim Hof Method, may influence the immune system's response to pathogens and inflammation. While more research is needed to fully understand the mechanisms involved, these findings hold promise for the potential role of breathwork in enhancing immune function.

Pain Perception and Tolerance:

The practice of breathwork has been investigated in the context of pain management. Research has shown that specific breathing techniques, combined with mindfulness, can reduce the perception of pain and improve pain tolerance. This has implications for individuals dealing with chronic pain conditions and may offer an adjunctive approach to pain management.

Cognitive Function:

Cognitive function and mental clarity can also be influenced by breathwork. Research indicates that mindful breathing practices can enhance cognitive performance, including attention, memory, and decision-making. These findings suggest that incorporating breathwork into daily routines may have cognitive benefits.

In conclusion, the growing body of research on breathwork and its effects on human physiology underscores its potential as a valuable tool for promoting health and well-being. From optimizing oxygenation and heart rate variability to regulating blood pressure and managing stress, breathwork offers a range of benefits that align with modern scientific understanding. Moreover, as research continues to uncover the mechanisms behind these effects, breathwork may find wider applications in healthcare, from improving cardiovascular health to enhancing immune function. Breathwork, once a practice rooted in tradition, is now firmly grounded in scientific exploration, offering individuals a pathway to better health and vitality through the simple act of conscious breathing.

Breathwork in Psychological Research

Breathwork in Psychological Research

Breathwork, a practice that involves conscious control and regulation of one's breath, has gained recognition in the field of psychological research for its profound effects on mental health, emotional well-being, and cognitive functioning. This essay explores the intersection of breathwork and psychological research, shedding light on how the simple act of mindful breathing can positively impact mental states and contribute to overall psychological well-being.

Stress Reduction and Anxiety Management:

Research in psychology has long established the relationship between stress and various mental health issues, including anxiety. Breathwork, specifically techniques like diaphragmatic breathing and mindful breathing, has been studied for its effectiveness in reducing stress and managing anxiety. When individuals engage in slow, deliberate breath control, it activates the body's relaxation response, reducing the production of stress hormones like cortisol. Studies have shown that regular breathwork practices can lead to a significant reduction in symptoms of anxiety disorders and stress-related conditions.

Emotional Regulation:

Emotion regulation is a critical aspect of mental health, and breathwork has emerged as a valuable tool in this regard. Psychological research has revealed that conscious breath control can influence the brain's emotional centers, helping individuals modulate their emotional responses. Deep breathing techniques, such as the 4-7-8 technique, have been shown to improve emotional regulation by calming the amygdala, the brain's "fear center." This research suggests that breathwork can assist individuals in managing emotional challenges, including anger, sadness, and frustration.

Mindfulness and Attention:

The practice of mindfulness involves paying focused attention to the present moment without judgment. Breathwork is an integral component of mindfulness-based interventions. Numerous studies have investigated the impact of mindfulness meditation, which incorporates breath awareness, on attention and cognitive functioning. Research has demonstrated that regular mindfulness practice can enhance attention span, cognitive flexibility, and working memory. This suggests that breathwork, as a central element of mindfulness, plays a crucial role in improving cognitive performance.

Post-Traumatic Stress Disorder (PTSD) and Trauma Recovery:

Post-traumatic stress disorder is a mental health condition that can result from exposure to traumatic events. Breathwork has been explored as a complementary approach to trauma recovery. Some research indicates that specific breathwork techniques, such as yoga breathing, may help individuals with PTSD manage their symptoms, including flashbacks and hyperarousal. While breathwork alone may not replace conventional trauma therapy, it can be a valuable adjunctive tool.

Depression and Mood Enhancement:

Depression is a prevalent mental health condition characterized by persistent low mood. Psychological studies have examined the potential of breathwork, particularly pranayama (breath control) from yoga traditions, to alleviate symptoms of depression. Controlled breathing exercises have been associated with increased production of mood-enhancing neurotransmitters like serotonin. Preliminary research suggests that breathwork may be a valuable component of a holistic approach to managing depression.

Sleep Quality and Insomnia:

Poor sleep and insomnia are common psychological complaints. Breathwork, especially relaxation-focused techniques, has been investigated for its ability to improve sleep quality. Research suggests that incorporating breathwork into bedtime routines can promote relaxation, reduce sleep disturbances, and enhance overall sleep patterns.

In conclusion, breathwork has found its place in psychological research as a versatile and accessible approach to improving mental health and well-being. The scientific evidence supports its efficacy in stress reduction, anxiety management, emotional regulation, attention enhancement, trauma recovery, mood enhancement, and sleep improvement. As researchers continue to explore the mechanisms underlying these effects, breathwork is likely to become an increasingly valuable tool in the field of psychology. Its integration into therapeutic practices and mental health interventions offers individuals a natural and holistic means of enhancing their psychological well-being. Breathwork serves as a powerful reminder that the breath, often taken for granted, can be a source of profound healing and resilience in the realm of mental health.

Breathwork for Specific Populations

Breathwork for Specific Populations

Breathwork is a versatile and accessible practice that offers a wide range of benefits, making it suitable for various populations, including children, athletes, individuals with chronic conditions, and those seeking to enhance their creativity. This essay explores how breathwork can be tailored to meet the unique needs and goals of these specific populations.

Children and Adolescents:

Breathwork techniques can be adapted to suit the needs of children and adolescents, helping them manage stress, anxiety, and emotional challenges. Simple breath awareness exercises, such as "belly breathing" or "balloon breath," can teach young individuals to regulate their emotions and improve focus. In educational settings, incorporating breathwork can create a calmer and more focused learning environment, potentially enhancing academic performance.

Athletes:

Breathwork has gained popularity among athletes for its potential to enhance physical and mental performance. Athletes often use breath control techniques, such as rhythmic breathing or breath-holding exercises, to optimize their oxygen intake and boost endurance. Additionally, breathwork can aid in managing pre-competition anxiety and improving recovery by promoting relaxation and reducing muscle tension.

Individuals with Chronic Conditions:

Breathwork can be particularly beneficial for individuals dealing with chronic health conditions such as asthma, chronic pain, or cardiovascular issues. Studies have shown that certain breathwork practices, like the Buteyko method, can help asthma patients reduce their reliance on medication and improve lung function. For those with chronic pain, breathwork can be integrated into pain management strategies to alleviate discomfort and promote relaxation.

Creativity and Artists:

Artists and creative individuals often turn to breathwork to enhance their creative processes. Techniques like "Holotropic Breathwork" or "circular breathing" are believed to expand consciousness and facilitate access to deep creativity. By altering one's state of consciousness through breathwork, artists may find new sources of inspiration and creative expression.

Pregnant Women and Childbirth:

Pregnant women can benefit from specific breathwork techniques designed to support them during childbirth. Lamaze, Hypnobirthing, and other childbirth education methods often incorporate breathwork to help manage pain and anxiety during labor. These techniques emphasize controlled and rhythmic breathing to promote relaxation and ease the birthing process.

Aging Population:

As individuals age, they may encounter challenges related to mobility, cognition, and overall well-being. Breathwork can be adapted to meet the needs of the aging population by focusing on gentle, seated breath exercises that promote relaxation, improve lung function, and enhance mental clarity. Regular breathwork practices can contribute to a sense of vitality and improved quality of life among seniors.

Individuals with Post-Traumatic Stress Disorder (PTSD):

Breathwork has shown promise as a complementary therapy for individuals with PTSD. Trauma-sensitive breathwork practices can help individuals with PTSD manage symptoms such as flashbacks, anxiety, and hyperarousal. These techniques prioritize safety, comfort, and gradual healing.

LGBTQ+ Community:

Breathwork can provide a safe space for self-exploration and self-acceptance within the LGBTQ+ community. It offers a means of releasing emotional stress, exploring gender and identity, and fostering a sense of belonging and self-love.

In conclusion, breathwork is a versatile practice that can be tailored to suit the unique needs and goals of specific populations. Whether it's helping children manage stress, enhancing athletic performance, aiding in chronic condition management, fueling creativity, supporting pregnant women during childbirth, promoting healthy aging, assisting individuals with PTSD, or providing a safe space for self-exploration within the LGBTQ+ community, breathwork offers a valuable tool for improving physical and mental well-being. By adapting breathwork techniques to the diverse needs of these populations, individuals can harness the power of the breath to lead healthier, more fulfilling lives.

Breathwork for Children

Breathwork for Children: Cultivating Calmness and Resilience

Breathwork, a practice that focuses on conscious control of the breath, has gained recognition for its numerous physical and mental health benefits. While often associated with adults, breathwork can also be a valuable tool for children, offering them ways to manage stress, enhance emotional well-being, and develop essential life skills. In this essay, we will explore the benefits of breathwork for children and discuss how it can be tailored to their unique needs.

Stress and Anxiety Management:

Children today face various stressors, including academic pressures, social challenges, and family issues. Breathwork provides children with practical tools to manage stress and anxiety effectively. Techniques like "belly breathing" or "balloon breath" encourage deep, diaphragmatic breathing, activating the body's relaxation response and reducing stress hormone levels. Regular practice of these techniques can help children build resilience and cope with everyday challenges more effectively.

Emotional Regulation:

One of the key benefits of breathwork for children is its ability to improve emotional regulation. Children often struggle with understanding and managing their emotions. Breath awareness exercises can teach them to connect with their feelings and respond to them in a healthy way. By recognizing the connection between their breath and emotions, children can learn to self-soothe and make more mindful choices in challenging situations.

Improved Concentration and Focus:

Children often find it challenging to stay focused for extended periods. Breathwork practices can enhance their concentration and attention span. Techniques like "box breathing," which involves inhaling, holding, exhaling, and holding the breath in equal counts, encourage mental clarity and enhance cognitive function. By incorporating breathwork into their daily routines, children can perform better academically and develop better problem-solving skills.

Emotional Resilience:

Breathwork can contribute to the development of emotional resilience in children. The practice teaches them to face difficult emotions and situations with equanimity. By embracing breath as a source of inner strength, children can build emotional resilience, enabling them to bounce back from adversity and navigate life's ups and downs more effectively.

Enhanced Self-Awareness:

Self-awareness is a crucial aspect of emotional intelligence. Breathwork helps children become more attuned to their bodies and emotions. They learn to recognize physical sensations associated with stress, anxiety, or excitement. This increased self-awareness allows them to address their emotional needs promptly and make healthier choices.

Better Sleep Patterns:

Children often struggle with sleep disturbances, which can negatively impact their overall well-being. Breathwork practices, such as "4-7-8 breathing," can promote relaxation and improve sleep quality. By engaging in calming breathwork exercises before bedtime, children can establish healthier sleep patterns and experience more restful nights.

Conflict Resolution and Empathy:

Breathwork can also foster positive social skills in children. By enhancing self-regulation and emotional awareness, it enables children to navigate conflicts more peacefully and develop empathy toward others. These skills are essential for building healthy relationships and a supportive social environment.

Fun and Playfulness:

Introducing breathwork to children in a playful and engaging manner is essential. Incorporating games, storytelling, or imaginative exercises into breathwork sessions can make the practice enjoyable for children. Creating a positive association with breathwork encourages them to embrace it as a valuable tool for self-care.

In conclusion, breathwork offers a range of benefits for children, including stress and anxiety management, emotional regulation, improved concentration, enhanced emotional resilience, self-awareness, better sleep patterns, conflict resolution skills, and a sense of playfulness. As children face various challenges and pressures in their lives, breathwork can empower them to build essential life skills that promote their physical and mental well-being. By introducing breathwork to children early on and making it an integral part of their daily routines, parents, educators, and caregivers can equip them with a valuable tool for navigating life's journey with greater ease and resilience.

Breathwork for the Elderly

Breathwork for the Elderly: A Path to Enhanced Well-being and Vitality

As we age, our bodies undergo various physiological changes, and maintaining good health becomes increasingly important. Breathwork, a practice centered on conscious control of the breath, offers a valuable tool for the elderly to promote physical fitness, emotional well-being, and overall vitality. In this essay, we will explore the benefits of breathwork for the elderly population and how it can contribute to a healthier and more fulfilling life in one's golden years.

Improved Respiratory Function:

With age, lung capacity tends to decrease, making it more challenging to breathe efficiently. Breathwork exercises focus on expanding lung capacity and strengthening respiratory muscles. Techniques like diaphragmatic breathing encourage deep inhalations, increasing oxygen intake and promoting better oxygenation of the body's tissues. Enhanced respiratory function can help seniors maintain their energy levels and reduce the risk of respiratory conditions.

Stress Reduction and Relaxation:

The elderly often face stressors related to health concerns, loneliness, or life transitions. Breathwork techniques, such as "relaxation breathing" or "counted breaths," can induce a relaxation response, reducing stress hormone levels and promoting a sense of calm. Regular practice of these techniques can help seniors manage stress and anxiety more effectively, leading to improved emotional well-being.

Pain Management:

Chronic pain is a common issue among the elderly. Breathwork offers a natural and drug-free approach to pain management. Techniques like "guided imagery" combined with breathwork can help seniors redirect their focus away from pain and reduce discomfort. Moreover, breathwork can facilitate the release of endorphins, the body's natural painkillers, providing relief from chronic pain conditions.

Enhanced Cardiovascular Health:

Cardiovascular health is a critical concern for seniors. Breathwork practices, such as "paced breathing," can have a positive impact on heart health. Controlled breathing helps regulate blood pressure, reduce heart rate, and improve circulation. These benefits contribute to a healthier cardiovascular system, reducing the risk of heart-related issues.

Increased Energy and Vitality:

Seniors often grapple with fatigue and a decline in overall energy levels. Breathwork exercises can help combat fatigue by increasing oxygen flow to the cells, enhancing energy production, and reducing feelings of exhaustion. Seniors who engage in breathwork may experience increased vitality, allowing them to participate in more activities and enjoy a higher quality of life.

Emotional Resilience and Well-being:

The elderly may face emotional challenges, such as grief, loss, or depression. Breathwork can aid in emotional resilience by helping seniors manage difficult emotions and improve their mood. Techniques like "square breathing" can stabilize emotions, fostering a greater sense of well-being and contentment.

Improved Cognitive Function:

Maintaining cognitive function is crucial for seniors to lead independent lives. Breathwork practices, particularly those that focus on deep, rhythmic breathing, can enhance brain oxygenation and cognitive performance. Improved oxygen supply to the brain supports better memory, mental clarity, and overall cognitive function.

Social Connection and Community:

Engaging in breathwork classes or group sessions can also provide seniors with opportunities for social interaction and a sense of community. These connections are essential for combating feelings of isolation and loneliness, which can negatively impact one's well-being.

In conclusion, breathwork is a versatile and accessible practice that can offer numerous benefits to the elderly population. By promoting improved respiratory function, stress reduction, pain management, enhanced cardiovascular health, increased energy, emotional resilience, cognitive function, and social connection, breathwork can contribute to a higher quality of life for seniors. As individuals age, maintaining physical fitness and emotional well-being becomes increasingly vital, and breathwork provides a valuable tool to achieve these goals. For the elderly, breathwork is not just a set of techniques; it is a path to enhanced well-being, vitality, and a more fulfilling life in the golden years.

Breathwork for Athletes

Breathwork for Athletes: Unlocking Peak Performance and Recovery

In the world of sports, athletes are continually seeking ways to gain an edge, whether it's in enhancing their physical abilities, speeding up recovery, or improving mental focus. Breathwork, a practice centered on conscious control of breathing, has emerged as a powerful tool for athletes looking to elevate their performance to new heights. In this essay, we will delve into the benefits of breathwork for athletes and how it can be integrated into training and competition strategies.

Enhanced Oxygen Utilization:

The primary goal of breathwork in athletic performance is to optimize oxygen utilization. Proper breathing techniques can increase oxygen intake, improve its delivery to muscles, and enhance utilization during exercise. This means more oxygen is available for energy production, reducing the risk of fatigue and allowing athletes to push their limits.

Improved Endurance:

For endurance athletes like marathon runners, cyclists, and triathletes, breath control is crucial. Breathwork techniques such as rhythmic breathing, where inhalations and exhalations are synchronized with stride or pedal cadence, help athletes maintain a steady pace and conserve energy. This can lead to significant improvements in endurance performance.

Stress Reduction:

Athletes often face high-stress levels during training and competition, which can negatively impact performance. Breathwork practices like diaphragmatic breathing and box breathing can activate the body's relaxation response, reducing stress hormone levels and calming the nervous system. This results in improved mental focus, better decision-making, and reduced performance anxiety.

Faster Recovery:

Recovery is a vital aspect of an athlete's training regimen. Proper recovery allows the body to repair and adapt to the demands of exercise. Breathwork aids in recovery by reducing muscle tension, promoting relaxation, and enhancing circulation. Techniques such as "recovery breathing" can accelerate the removal of metabolic waste products, leading to quicker recovery between workouts or competitions.

Injury Prevention:

Breathwork can contribute to injury prevention by increasing body awareness. Athletes who practice breathwork develop better proprioception, which is the ability to sense the position and movement of their bodies. Improved body awareness can help athletes avoid overuse injuries and maintain proper form during exercise.

Mental Toughness:

Success in sports often depends on mental resilience and the ability to push through physical discomfort. Breathwork techniques, like breath holds or progressive muscle relaxation, can train athletes to tolerate discomfort and maintain focus under pressure. This mental toughness can make a significant difference in competition.

Rehabilitation and Injury Management:

Athletes recovering from injuries can benefit from breathwork as part of their rehabilitation process. Controlled breathing can help alleviate pain, reduce muscle tension around injured areas, and improve circulation to promote healing. It also allows athletes to maintain some level of physical conditioning while recovering.

Pre-Competition Preparation:

Breathwork serves as an essential tool in pre-competition rituals. Athletes can use specific breathwork techniques to calm nerves, increase confidence, and mentally prepare for the challenges ahead. Visualization combined with controlled breathing can create a mental state conducive to peak performance.

Post-Competition Recovery:

After a demanding competition, athletes can use breathwork to accelerate recovery and reduce the risk of post-competition stress or burnout. Relaxation and deep breathing can help athletes unwind and transition from the heightened state of competition to a state of rest and recovery.

Team Building and Cohesion:

Breathwork can also be used as a team-building exercise. Group breathwork sessions can foster a sense of cohesion among teammates, improve communication, and create a supportive atmosphere within the team.

In conclusion, breathwork is a versatile and powerful tool for athletes of all levels. Its ability to enhance oxygen utilization, improve endurance, reduce stress, speed up recovery, prevent injuries, build mental toughness, aid in rehabilitation, and prepare athletes for competition makes it a valuable addition to any training regimen. Athletes who incorporate breathwork into their routines may find themselves achieving new levels of performance, both physically and mentally. In the world of sports, where every fraction of a second or inch can make a difference, breathwork is proving to be a game-changer, unlocking the potential for peak performance and recovery.

Have Questions / Comments?

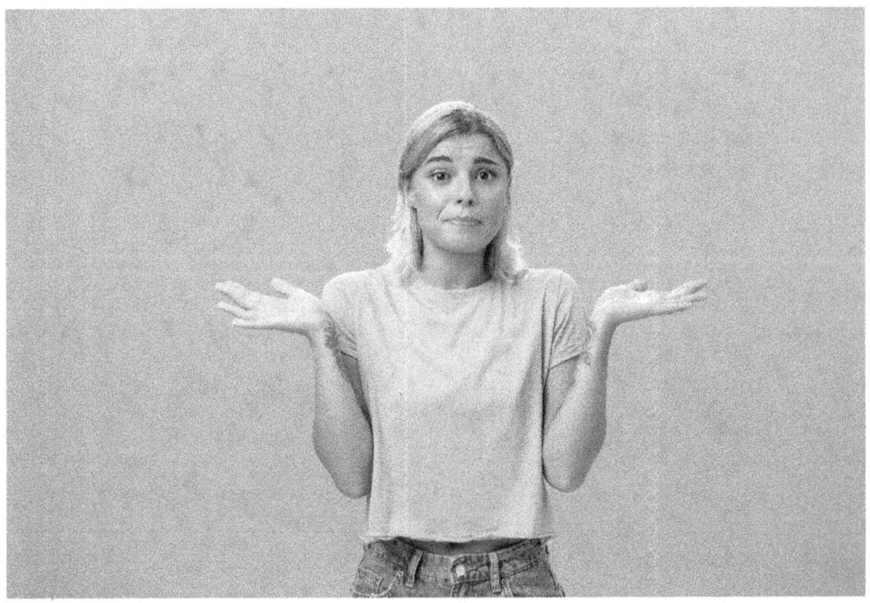

This book was designed to cover as much as possible but I know I have probably missed something, or some new amazing discovery that has just come out.

If you notice something missing or have a question that I failed to answer, please get in touch and let me know. If I can, I will email you an answer and also update the book so others can also benefit from it.

Thanks For Being Awesome :)

Submit Your Questions / Comments At:

https://xspurts.com/posts/questions

Get Another Book Free

We love writing and have produced a huge number of books.

For being one of our amazing readers, we would love to offer you another book we have created, 100% free.

To claim this limited time special offer, simply go to the site below and enter your name and email address.

You will then receive one of my great books, direct to your email account, 100% free!

https://xspurts.com/posts/free-book-offer